# Sexually Transmitted Diseases

Leanne Currie-McGhee

## Diseases and Disorders

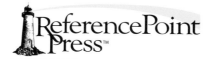

ReferencePoint Press™

San Diego, CA

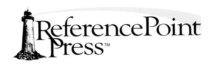

© 2009 ReferencePoint Press, Inc.

**For more information, contact:**
ReferencePoint Press, Inc.
PO Box 27779
San Diego, CA 92198
www. ReferencePointPress.com

Picture credits:
Maury Aaseng: 31–35, 50–53, 67–70, 84–88
AP Images: 15
Landov: 11

LIBRARY OF CONGRESS CATALOGING-IN-PUBLICATION DATA

Currie-McGhee, (Leanne)
  Sexually Transmitted Diseases / by Leanne Currie-McGhee.
    p. cm. — (Compact research series)
  Includes bibliographical references and index.
  ISBN-13: 978-1-60152-045-6 (hardback)
  ISBN-10: 1-60152-045-X (hardback)
  1. Sexually transmitted diseases. I. Title.
  RA644.V4C77 2008
  614.5'47— dc22

                                                          2008012554

# Conte

# Foreword

As modern civilization continues to evolve, its ability to create, store, distribute, and access information expands exponentially. The explosion of information from all media continues to increase at a phenomenal rate. By 2020 some experts predict the worldwide information base will double every 73 days. While access to diverse sources of information and perspectives is paramount to any democratic society, information alone cannot help people gain knowledge and understanding. Information must be organized and presented clearly and succinctly in order to be understood. The challenge in the digital age becomes not the creation of information, but how best to sort, organize, enhance, and present information.

ReferencePoint Press developed the *Compact Research* series with this challenge of the information age in mind. More than any other subject area today, researching current issues can yield vast, diverse, and unqualified information that can be intimidating and overwhelming for even the most advanced and motivated researcher. The *Compact Research* series offers a compact, relevant, intelligent, and conveniently organized collection of information covering a variety of current topics ranging from illegal immigration and methamphetamine to diseases such as anorexia and meningitis.

The series focuses on three types of information: objective single-author narratives, opinion-based primary source quotations, and facts and statistics. The clearly written objective narratives provide context and reliable background information. Primary source quotes are carefully selected and cited, exposing the reader to differing points of view. And facts and statistics sections aid the reader in evaluating perspectives. Presenting these key types of information creates a richer, more balanced learning experience.

For better understanding and convenience, the series enhances information by organizing it into narrower topics and adding design features that make it easy for a reader to identify desired content. For example, in *Compact Research: Illegal Immigration*, a chapter covering the economic impact of illegal immigration has an objective narrative explaining the various ways the economy is impacted, a balanced section of numerous primary source quotes on the topic, followed by facts and full-color illustrations to encourage evaluation of contrasting perspectives.

The ancient Roman philosopher Lucius Annaeus Seneca wrote, "It is quality rather than quantity that matters." More than just a collection of content, the *Compact Research* series is simply committed to creating, finding, organizing, and presenting the most relevant and appropriate amount of information on a current topic in a user-friendly style that invites, intrigues, and fosters understanding.

# Sexually Transmitted Diseases at a Glance

## Types of Disease

Sexually transmitted diseases (STDs) can be bacterial, viral, or parasitic. Viral STDs are incurable, although the body is able to rid itself of some viral infections on its own. Among the most common STDs are chlamydia, syphilis, gonorrhea, and herpes.

## Transmission

STDs are transmitted via oral, vaginal, or anal sexual contact between two people. Additionally, some STDs can be transmitted through blood contact and from a pregnant woman to her unborn child.

## Main Symptoms

Symptoms for STDs vary depending on the STD. Typical symptoms include sores on the genitals, burning during urination, and itching in the genitals. Certain STDs, such as chlamydia, often do not have symptoms.

## Severe Consequences

If left untreated, most STDs can result in serious health problems including cervical cancer, liver damage, infertility, and, in some cases, death.

## Treatment

Bacterial STDs can be cured with antibiotics. Parasitic STDs can typically be cured with topical medications. Viral STDs cannot be cured by treatment, but the symptoms and serious damage of these diseases can be mitigated with different types of medications.

## People Most at Risk

STDs affect men and women of all races and socioeconomic statuses. However, STDs disproportionately affect women, infants of infected mothers, and adolescents.

## Prevention

The most effective way a person can avoid contracting an STD is by abstaining from sex. Using a latex condom during sex is also effective at reducing the chances of contracting an STD.

## Epidemics

Sub-Saharan Africa is suffering from a human immunodeficiency virus (HIV) epidemic. In 2007 an estimated 22.5 million people were living with HIV, and an estimated 1.6 million people in that region died from acquired immunodeficiency syndrome (AIDS). The epidemic has led to millions of orphans, food shortages, and economic instability.

## Medical Research

In the past century, successful medical research has led to vaccines for hepatitis B (HBV) and certain strains of human papillomavirus (HPV); aggressive treatments for HIV; rapid tests for STDs; and cures for syphilis, chlamydia, and gonorrhea.

# Overview

**" Sex—the simple act of human coupling that is essential to our futures—is soaked with risks."**

—Gerald N. Callahan, *Infection: The Uninvited Universe.*

Sexually transmitted diseases, or STDs, are defined as infections transmitted via sexual contact between two people. The sexual contact may be in the form of vaginal, anal, or oral sex between a woman and a man, a man and a man, or a woman and a woman. Some STDs can also be transmitted nonsexually, such as through blood contact or when an infected pregnant woman passes the infection to her unborn child.

More than half of all people will be infected with an STD at some point in their lives. Worldwide, nearly a million people acquire one of the more than 30 different types of STDs every day. According to the National Institute of Allergy and Infectious Diseases (NIAID), STDs are among the most common infectious diseases in the United States. Common STDs include bacterial STDs such as chlamydia, gonorrhea, and syphilis; parasitic STDs such as pubic lice and trichomoniasis; and viral STDs such as herpes, human papillomavirus (HPV), hepatitis B (HBV), and human immunodeficiency virus (HIV)/acquired immunodeficiency syndrome (AIDS).

Often STDs are left untreated because people do not realize they have a disease. This is because many STDs are not accompanied with symptoms. Unfortunately, untreated STDs can result in serious physical damage. For example, Kim Bresnehan of the United Kingdom never knew she had had an attack of chlamydia until she experienced its aftereffects years later.

Bresnehan got married in her 20s and discovered she could not conceive a child. Bresnehan went to a doctor and learned that her fallopian tubes had been damaged from an earlier episode with chlamydia. She likely contracted the STD as a teenager and never knew it.

"Every time I went to the family planning clinic to get a new prescription for the Pill, they'd tell me: 'If you get sick, come and see us and we'll clear it up,'" Bresnehan says of her teenage years. "But I wasn't worried. I was monogamous and my boyfriends did not have any symptoms."[1] She never felt sick and did not return to the clinic. The result was that undiagnosed chlamydia damaged her reproductive system, leaving her infertile.

In addition to infertility, untreated STDs can lead to cervical cancer, neurological damage, and liver cancer. Some STDs, such as HBV and HIV/AIDS, can lead to complications that result in death. For this reason, health professionals urge all sexually active people to get regularly tested for STDs.

## STDs Past and Present

In the 1960s, if a person was diagnosed with an STD and had access to medical care, he or she could easily be treated. At the time, gonorrhea and syphilis—bacterial STDs—were the most common STDs. Once diagnosed, both of these STDs could be cured with antibiotics.

The impact of STDs has significantly changed since that time. In 1976 a new bacterial STD, chlamydia, was discovered. Today, chlamydia affects more than 3 million people in the United States each year. Another prevalent viral STD, genital herpes, became prevalent in the 1980s. Following that, HIV, one of the deadliest STDs, was identified. Today, there are over 30 known STDs.

> **More than half of all people will be infected with an STD at some point in their lives.**

The STDs discovered in the past 50 years are more difficult to treat than the ones discovered previously. HPV, HIV, genital herpes, and HBV are incurable. Additionally, HPV, HBV, and HIV can be fatal. Two strains of HPV, which is the most common viral STD, were identified as the cause of 70 percent of cervical cancer in women. Hepatitis B can lead to liver cancer. HIV can develop into AIDS, which killed approximately 2.1 million people in 2007.

## Who Is Affected by STDS?

STDs do not discriminate. A person of any gender, sexual orientation, race, or socioeconomic class is at risk for an STD if he or she engages in any type of sexual relations. According to the World Health Organization (WHO), approximately 340 million new cases of bacterial and parasitic STDs occur throughout the year. Additionally, according to WHO, viral STDs infect millions of people worldwide each year.

Certain people are more susceptible to contracting an STD than others. For both biological and societal reasons, women are more susceptible than men to STDs. In many parts of the world, women are not empowered to make their own sexual decisions. For example, if their husbands refuse to use a condom during sex, even if the men are infected with an STD, women still must have sex with their husbands.

Also for biological and societal reasons, teenagers are more susceptible to STDs. Teenagers' immune systems are not mature, and so they are more susceptible to infections. Also, teenagers are often more sexually active than older adults and lack STD knowledge.

> A person of any gender, sexual orientation, race, or socio-economic class is at risk for an STD if he or she engages in any type of sexual relations.

People in certain areas of the world are more at risk for contracting an STD. In countries where it is difficult to access health care, people are susceptible to contracting and passing on STDs. For example, in sub-Saharan Africa, HIV has become an epidemic; it affects over 20 percent of the population in some countries. Because of the lack of access to health care, many infected people are not diagnosed and continue to pass the disease to sexual partners. Infected pregnant women are unable to get treatment, and so they pass the disease on to their unborn children.

## What Behaviors Increase STD Risk?

Certain behaviors increase a person's risk of contracting an STD. Unprotected sex with multiple partners and sharing needles during drug use are the two most common risky behaviors. For this reason, prostitutes and

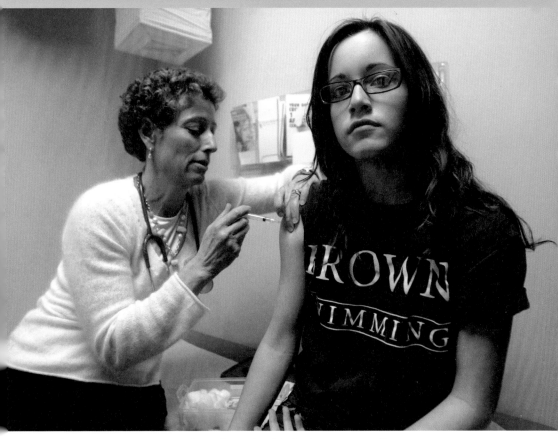

*This girl, 15, receives a shot of Gardasil. The human papillomavirus vaccine became available in 2006. The FDA reported that in women who had not already been infected, Gardasil was nearly 100 percent effective in preventing precancerous cervical lesions, precancerous vaginal and vulvar lesions, and genital warts caused by infection of the four types of HPV the vaccine protects against.*

substance abusers are among people who are at high risk for contracting an STD.

For example, India's prostitutes have an estimated 10 to 20 percent HIV prevalence rate due to their behavior. Kamathipura, a district in Mumbai, India, has more than 60,000 prostitutes. These prostitutes, mainly women, receive approximately $1.50 (U.S. dollars) for sex. In addition to having multiple sexual partners, these women increase their STD risk by having sex without a condom. They do this because their male clients pay more for sex without condoms. The men do not consider having unprotected sex a health risk. "Most of the men I spoke to as they were visiting brothels said they saw no relationship between wearing a condom and preventing HIV and AIDS," *Frontline* producer and reporter Raney Aronson says regarding her interviews with sex workers and their clients throughout India. "So they saw no compelling reason to wear them."[2]

> By the end of 2005, approximately 4 million . . . injecting drug users were infected with HIV.

Injecting drug users' behavior also results in a high prevalence rate of HIV. Sharing syringes is an easy way to transmit blood-borne viruses such as HIV. Some studies have found that the sharing of needles is three times more likely to transmit HIV than sexual intercourse. The United Nations estimates that there were 13.2 million injecting drug users globally at the end of 2003, and by the end of 2005, approximately 4 million of these injecting drug users were infected with HIV.

## What Are the Dangers of STDs?

For those who get STDs, serious health problems can result. Initially, many STDs begin with no symptoms. However, if left undiagnosed and untreated, STDs can result in severe and chronic health problems. "The big deal [about STDs] is HIV severely disrupts the immune system and can kill; human papilloma virus can give you cancer; chlamydia can make you sterile; syphilis can cause brain disease and can cause congenital malformations—and that's just a sample,"[3] explains Peter Borriello, director of the United Kingdom Health Protection Agency's Centre for Infections.

Bacterial STDs, some of the most common being syphilis, chlamydia, and gonorrhea, are curable if discovered early. However, if left untreated, these three can have devastating results such as pelvic inflammatory disease (PID) in women and epididymitis in men. Epididymitis is an inflammation of the epididymis, the coiled tube at the back of the testicle that stores and carries sperm. Both men and women can suffer from neurological, cardiovascular, and organ damage, and even death.

Viral STDs, such as genital herpes, HBV, HPV, and HIV, are not curable and can produce lifelong effects. A person infected with herpes will likely experience outbreaks of genital blisters and sores for the rest of his or her life. HBV can result in severe liver disease, including cirrhosis and liver cancer. HPV may lead to cervical cancer and genital warts. HIV is the most feared viral STD, as it is incurable and, if untreated, quickly becomes AIDS. A person with AIDS has a severely weakened immune system and is at risk of dying from opportunistic infections. These are infections that typically do not cause disease in a person with a healthy immune system.

In addition to the physical problems, people with STDs also suffer psychological issues. This is because of the stigma associated with STDs. Many people with STDs, in particular HIV, are discriminated against or looked down upon by others. Because of this discrimination, it is difficult for many infected people to talk about their STDs. Many avoid dating or getting into romantic relationships because they do not want to have to discuss their STDs. This can lead to loneliness and depression.

## Failing Economies

Untreated STDs have led to major economic problems in developing countries. According to the WHO, STDs account for 17 percent of economic losses caused by ill health in developing countries. These countries are losing workers due to illness and deaths from STDs. Those who cannot work because of ill health cannot afford to care for their families. The governments must direct their limited resources to providing health care and food to the ill and their families.

Sub-Saharan Africa has born the major brunt of STDs, particularly AIDS. Its countries' governments cannot afford to care for the sick. Nearly two-thirds of all HIV-positive people live in this area, although it contains little more than 10 percent of the world's population. In the same region, the

> " Viral STDs, such as genital herpes, HBV, HPV, and HIV, are not curable and can produce lifelong effects. "

medical costs of AIDS, not including antiretroviral therapy, have been estimated at about $30 per year for every person infected. Overall, public health spending is less than $10 per year per individual for most African countries.

The result of the monetary costs of STDS and the loss of workers due to ill health is that sub-Saharan African countries are experiencing poverty, declines in their average life expectancies, labor shortages, less educated people, millions of orphaned children, and even food shortages. "Our fields are idle because there is nobody to work them," says Toby Solomon, commisioner for the Nsanje district in Malawi. "We don't have machinery for farming, we only have manpower—if we are sick, or spend our time looking after family members who are sick, we have no time to spend working in the fields."[4]

## Can Changes in Behavior Prevent STDs?

One of the ways to prevent STDs and decrease their impact on the world is to teach people how to lower their risk of infection. Both national health agencies such as the U.S. Centers for Disease Control (CDC) and the international health agencies such as WHO focus on teaching people the ABC message. The ABC message is to Abstain, Be faithful, and use Condoms.

Programs using the ABC message stress that the most effective way to prevent infection from an STD is to abstain from sex. However, if a person chooses to have sex, the best way to reduce his or her risk is to have sex only in a monogamous relationship and to use latex condoms during sex. Latex condoms are effective at preventing STDs. Prevention programs also focus on getting people tested for STDs so that they can get treated and not infect others. Programs also encourage infected people to notify their sexual partners so that their partners can get tested, treated if necessary, and prevent themselves from infecting others.

> **The ABC message is to Abstain, Be faithful, and use Condoms.**

The CDC has found that its U.S. prevention programs are successful. For example, Project Respect involved nearly 6,000 heterosexual men and women who attended STD clinics in five U.S. cities. Project Respect counselors talked with patients, rather than lectured them, in order to understand their lifestyles. Based on discussions, counselors and patients worked together to make an STD risk-reduction plan. In some cases this included abstinence, and in others the plan included condom use. The CDC found that this method resulted in a 20 percent decrease in new STDs among study participants.

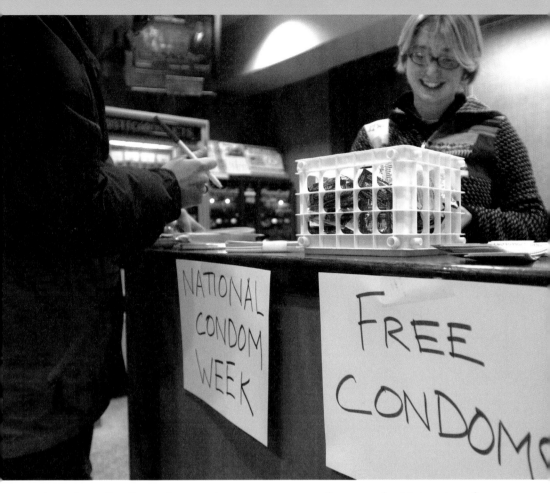

*A student distributes free condoms to promote safe sex at the University of Wisconsin in Madison. For sexually active people, condom use can protect against many diseases.*

## Prevention Methods for Those Most at Risk

Despite prevention programs, many people, often those most at risk, do not change their sexual behavior. This is because it is difficult for them to implement changes in their lifestyles. For example, sex workers, people who have sex with others for money, often do not use condoms because they do not have access to them, or clients refuse to pay for and use them.

To convince more sex workers to use condoms, governments and health agencies have implemented innovative prevention programs. For example, Thailand's government implemented a condom use program among sex workers. Although prostitution is illegal in Thailand, the government has worked with brothel owners to enforce 100 percent condom use among its prostitutes. The government distributes condoms free to brothels, and the brothel owners ensure that their sex workers insist that clients use the condoms. To be certain this occurs, government inspectors pose as clients to check the brothels.

> " People who have sex with others for money often do not use condoms because they do not have access to them, or clients refuse to pay for and use them. "

South Africa has also implemented programs to target high-risk populations such as migrant workers, men who work away from their families and live in hostels, and sex workers, whom migrant workers often turn to for sex. A medical clinic near a South African mining community with several single-sex mining hostels offered free STD prevention and treatment services to the nearby sex workers. During the study of this medical clinic, women sex workers' rates of gonorrheal infection dropped from 15 percent to 8 percent by their third clinic visit. Over the same period, the prevalence of gonorrhea or chlamydia among male migrant workers decreased from 11 percent to 6 percent. These successes have led to similar programs throughout the world.

## Barriers to Prevention

Despite prevention programs, both established and new, major barriers still prevent many people from reducing their chances of contracting STDs. Worldwide, of those who are at risk of contracting HIV, fewer than one in five has access to prevention programs. As a result, many people do not understand what they can do to reduce their risk. For example, a 2004 WHO study found that in Moldova, the Ukraine, and Uzbekistan, more than three-fourths of women could not list the three methods to prevent AIDS—abstinence, condoms, and an exclusive relationship with a faithful partner.

Another issue with prevention programs is people's reluctance to change their sexual practices. Some people learn about how to prevent STDs but do not use their knowledge. In the United States, Jaime knew that unprotected sex could lead to sexually transmitted diseases or pregnancy. However, when she chose to have sex with her new boyfriend, she did so unprotected. "I guess it was embarrassment," she says. "I waited for him to say something about it, and since he didn't, I didn't either."[5]

A lack of sex education curriculum might also increase risks of contracting an STD. For example, in India 44 percent of reported AIDS cases occur among 15- to 29-year-olds. However, great controversy erupted when the government rolled out a national sex education program to be taught in the schools. Nasratullah Afandi of Jamaat-e-Islami Hind, an Islamic cultural organization, was against the program. He stated, "Sex is instinctive. It is not necessary to teach children about it."[6] In Delhi, the sex education program never reached any schools. Rina Ray, education secretary in the local government, said that the Delhi school system would introduce its own course that would emphasize life skills like nutrition, decision making, and communicating with one's parents. The Delhi program would not include information about sex and AIDS.

## Can Science Eliminate STDs?

In addition to preventing STDs with behavior modification, both health officials and medical professionals believe that scientific means are necessary to reduce and eventually eliminate STDs. In the past decade, people, nongovernmental organizations (NGOs), governments, and corporations have funded STD scientific research programs with billions of dollars in hope of finding medical ways to prevent and cure STDs. With this funding, researchers have made major scientific leaps.

Recent medical research has resulted in easier and more accurate testing of STDs, including chlamydia, HPV, and HIV. A person who is diagnosed quickly has the chance of a cure in certain cases and knows to avoid infecting others. Other advances include the development of the HBV and HPV vaccines. A person who receives these vaccines has very little chance of contracting HBV and the sexual strains of HPV. In addition, medical advances have led to treatments of all STDs.

> " Recent medical research has resulted in easier and more accurate testing of STDs, including chlamydia, HPV, and HIV. "

One of the main supporters of U.S. STD research is the U.S. National Institutes of Health. This governmental organization provides leadership and funding for scientific research of treatments and medical ways to prevent STDs. Its research includes clinical trials of various medications and treatments for all types of STDs. In 2008, examples of ongoing clinical trials included testing a genital herpes vaccine for women, new drug therapies for people infected with chronic hepatitis B, and new types of gels for women to prevent STD infections.

## Surviving with an STD

Because of the scientific breakthroughs, more people have been cured of STDs. For people with incurable STDs, medical breakthroughs have enabled them to live longer and more active lives. For example, HIV is no longer the death sentence it was in the 1980s. Today a person with HIV who takes antiretroviral drugs (ARVs) may live for decades.

Peter Dobson, a computer scientist from Los Angeles, is one of millions who have benefited from ARVs. Dobson discovered in the 1980s that he was infected with HIV. He expected to die just like many of his friends who had already died from AIDS. However, the first anti-HIV medication became available, and he took it. Since then he has continued to take the improved drugs that scientific research has developed in the last two decades.

Because of the medications, Dobson has been healthy enough to work and help others who have HIV. "Medical research saved my life," Dobson says. "But I am looking for even better HIV drugs. And—a cure would be nice."[7] The health and scientific communities hope and work for the same, not only for HIV but all STDs.

# What Are Sexually Transmitted Diseases?

"The microbes that cause sexually transmitted diseases are equal opportunity bugs. They don't care if you are white or black, rich or poor, educated or illiterate, happy or sad. If you're a warm body, you'll do."

—Student Health Services of the University of North Carolina at Greensboro.

Sexually transmitted diseases (STDs) and sexually transmitted infections (STIs) infect over a million people worldwide each day. STDs and STIs are primarily sexually transmitted and can result in serious damage to a person's physical health. The extent of the damage depends on whether an STI develops into an STD, what STD a person has contracted, how quickly he or she is diagnosed, and what type of treatment the person has access to.

STDs and STIs are often used interchangeably, but the two are not the same. A person is infected with an STI when a sexually transmitted organism has invaded his or her body. However, the organism may not develop into a disease. Sometimes the body is able to rid itself of the infection before it turns into a disease. This occasionally occurs with organisms that cause HPV or HBV. Sometimes they enter the body, but the body fights them off before they turn into an STD. However, most STIs do become STDs.

## What Are Bacterial STDs?

STDs are causes by three types of organisms: bacteria, parasites, and viruses. Of these, STDs caused by bacteria are the most common.

Bacteria are living microscopic germs that usually consist of a single cell. Bacterial organisms thrive in a moist and warm environment, such as the body's tissues, and die quickly outside of this environment. For this reason, bacterial STDs are passed through sexual contact, but cannot be passed through sharing of towels and clothes. Once inside the body, these germs cling together and feed off the host body.

> **All bacterial STDs are curable if treatment is sought.**

Three of the most common bacterial STDs are chlamydia, gonorrhea, and syphilis. Chlamydia is the most prevalent and, according to 2006 estimates by the CDC, affects nearly 3 million Americans a year. In 2006 the CDC also estimated that more than 700,000 people in the United States were newly infected with gonorrhea. Syphilis cases had significantly decreased in the late 1990s, down to 5,979 in the United States by the year 2000. However, by 2006 its numbers had increased to 36,935 reported cases.

These three STDs can cause major damage to the body if left untreated. However, all bacterial STDs are curable if treatment is sought. Antibiotics can easily clear up these diseases.

## What Are Parasitic STDs?

Parasitic STDs are caused by parasites, small animals that get nourishment from the person they infect. STD parasites prefer to reside in the person's pubic area. They are transmitted through contact with sexual partners' genital areas.

The most common parasitic STD is trichomoniasis. According to the NIAD, 170 million people are affected worldwide. Trichomoniasis is caused by the single-celled protozoan parasite *Trichomonas vaginalis* that is microscopic in size. The trichomoniasis parasite is sexually transmitted through penis-to-vagina intercourse or vulva-to-vulva contact with an infected partner. Women can become infected with the disease from infected men or women, but men typically can only get it from infected women. Trichomoniasis can usually be cured with prescription drugs given by mouth in a single dose.

Another common parasitic STD is pubic lice, also known as crabs. Pubic lice are insects found in the genital areas of people and, unlike the *Trichomonas* protozoan parasites, can be seen by the naked eye. Pubic lice are typically spread through sexual contact. Although it occurs rarely, pubic lice also can be spread through contact with an infected person's bed linens, towels, or clothes. A person can easily be cured of pubic lice with a lice-killing shampoo that is available at drug stores without a prescription.

## What Are Viral STDs?

The most serious STDs are those caused by viruses. Viruses are complex molecules that attach to the outer surface of a cell and then get inside the cell. Once inside the cell, the molecules force the cell to make new viral proteins and new copies of the virus's genes. The "hijacked" cell then infects other cells. Examples of common viral STDs are HIV, hepatitis B (HBV), human papillomavirus (HPV) and genital herpes.

Viral STDs are passed through bodily fluids during anal, oral, or vaginal sex. Many viral STDs can be passed through blood contact, such as through sharing needles. Viral STDs affect millions of people, including approximately 33.2 million people currently living with HIV, 400 million with chronic hepatitis B, and 86 million with genital herpes.

Viral STDs are generally considered more dangerous than bacterial and parasitic STDs. This is because viral STDs cannot be cured through medical treatment. Although treatments are available to mitigate symptoms, a person who gets genital herpes or HIV will be infected for life. Some viral STDs, such as HPV and hepatitis B, may clear up on their own. Viral STDs are also considered more dangerous than the other STD categories because a person with a viral STD has a greater chance of developing a serious ailment such as liver cancer in the case of hepatitis B, cervical cancer with HPV, and opportunistic infections with HIV/AIDS.

> " Viral STDs are generally considered more dangerous than bacterial and parasitic STDs. This is because viral STDs cannot be cured through medical treatment. "

## How Are STDs Spread?

STDs are most commonly spread by sexual contact between two people. An infected person can spread an STD through body fluids such as semen, vaginal fluids, and blood. The sexual contact may be in the form of vaginal, anal, or oral sex. This can be between a woman and a man, a man and a man, or a woman and a woman. Anyone who is having any type of sexual relations is at risk of becoming infected with an STD.

Most STDs cannot be spread through casual contact such as with toilet seats, swimming pools, hot tubs, shared clothing, door knobs, or eating utensils. However, syphilis can be transmitted by direct contact with the open sores. In this case, kissing another person where they have an open sore can spread the disease. And herpes can invade the body anywhere an open herpes sore comes in contact with a break in the skin.

Some STDs, such as HIV, can also be transmitted by blood contact. People can transfer HIV by sharing needles or when an infected person's blood comes in contact with an open cut on an uninfected person. Many STDs can be passed from an infected woman to her fetus, newborn, or infant. Some STDs can infect the fetus during its development. Other STDs are transmitted from an infected mother to her child as the infant passes through the birth canal. HIV, unlike other STDs, can also infect a child through the mother's breast milk.

> " Most STDs cannot be spread [from person to person] through casual contact. "

Jasmine, an American fifth grader, was born with HIV. "I got it from my mom. My dad also had HIV," Jasmine explains. "I get scared sometimes that my mom might die. My dad died when I was four years old, and it's been me and my mom since then. My mom has been giving me my medicine since the day I was born."[8]

## How Prevalent Are STDS?

STDs are a worldwide problem. According to the World Health Organization (WHO), over 340 million people are infected with STDs each year. Certain areas of the world are more impacted than others. Generally, poorer countries have higher STD prevalence rates due to lack of access to prevention programs, health care, and treatment.

Sub-Saharan Africa is a region where people are at great risk for STDs. People in this region are estimated to account for 11 to 35 percent of the world's new cases of curable STDs. As for incurable STDs, according to a 2006 WHO report, between 10 and 80 percent of women and between 10 and 50 percent of men in this region are infected with genital herpes. Sub-Saharan Africa also bears most of the burden of HIV/AIDS with 22.5 million HIV-positive people, over 60 percent of the worldwide cases. The main reason is that people in this region are poor and lack access to health care, where they could be diagnosed, treated, and in some cases, cured of STDs.

> " **Sub-Saharan Africa also bears most of the burden of HIV/AIDS with 22.5 million HIV-positive people, over 60 percent of the worldwide cases.** "

Wealthier nations, however, are not immune to STDs. In fact, more than one in five adults in the United States is currently living with a viral STD, which, according to the American Social Health Association, is the highest infection rate of any industrialized country. Nineteen million Americans become newly infected with an STD each year. The CDC reports that certain STD rates are rising in the United States, including chlamydia, HPV, and syphilis. A major reason for this rise is that despite prevention programs, people still do not believe they are at risk for STDs and do not practice safe sex.

## Brunt of Disease Affects Women

Although both men and women around the world are susceptible to STDs, women are more at risk than men. Statistics show that more women than men are infected with many of the most common STDs. In the United States, among the chlamydia diagnoses reported in 2006, the male to female ratio was 253,236 to 777,675. According to Avert, an international AIDS charity, in 2007 women made up 50 percent of all adults living with HIV worldwide, a significant increase from when HIV was first discovered. In the first years of HIV, it mainly affected homosexual males and very few women. Then HIV crossed over to heterosexuals. Once this occurred, the number of female cases increased at a greater rate than male cases. In some parts of the world, women now have overtaken men in the number of AIDS cases. For example, in sub-Saharan Africa women account for 61 percent of the area's HIV cases.

One reason for these statistics is that women are biologically more at risk for an STD than men because a woman has more genital surface exposed during sex. Additionally, this surface is more susceptible to small tears than men's. STD bacteria and viruses can infect the body through these tears.

In certain parts of the world, society and culture expose women to STDs. In certain countries women's social status puts them under the power of men. The men make all the decisions, including those regarding sex. For example, in male-dominant societies a woman often cannot say no to sex or ask her partner to use a condom. She can be forced to have unprotected sex.

In Tamilnadu, India, P. Kousalya, president of the Positive Women's Network, an organization supporting HIV-positive women, contracted HIV from nonconsensual sex with her husband. "After my marriage my husband forced me to have sex with him, even though I was unwilling and I spent a lot of time crying unseen in my room," says Kousalya. "I spent three months with my husband's family, after which I fell sick along with my husband. My husband tested HIV positive when he went for a checkup. My entire family knew his status, except me. Later, I found out. AIDS!"[9]

> " **In male-dominant societies a woman often cannot say no to sex or ask her partner to use a condom.** "

## Teens and Susceptibility

Young adults, particularly teenagers, are another subgroup especially at risk for STDs. According to the Centers for Disease Control, estimates suggest that while 15- to 24-year-olds represent 25 percent of the sexually active population, the same group acquires nearly half of all new STDs. The reasons for this are due both to biology and behavior.

Biologically, young people have immature immune systems. This makes them less able to fight off infections such as STDs. Additionally, younger women are more likely than adult women to experience tearing during intercourse. Also, the cervix of an adolescent female is covered with cells that are especially susceptible to STDs.

Behaviors also put both male and female teenagers more at risk for STDs than adults. One behavior that puts younger adults at risk is making sexual decisions when under the influence of drugs or alcohol. Research has linked adolescent alcohol use to high-risk sex, which includes sex with multiple partners and unprotected sex. Another high-risk behavior is that young adults often do not use condoms. According to a 2006 *USA Today* survey, 53 percent of sexually active American male teenagers said they do not always use a condom. Among the sexually active girls, nearly two-thirds said they do not always use a condom.

> **Research has linked adolescent alcohol use to high-risk sex, which includes sex with multiple partners and unprotected sex.**

Holly Becker was 17 years old when she decided to have sex with her boyfriend, Derek. He told her that he had tested negative for any STDs. She still asked him to wear a condom. "A little while into the sex, I could tell he hadn't put on a condom," writes Becker. "I knew then that I'd made a mistake, but I didn't stop him. I was embarrassed and afraid of being rejected."[10] Soon after, Becker discovered she was infected with genital herpes, a lifelong disease.

Unless a cure for herpes is found, Becker must deal with both the physical and emotional damage of living with an STD for the rest of her life. She and millions of people infected with an STD around the world live in the hope that cures or treatments for their STDs will be soon discovered. Until that occurs, they must deal with the daily impact of STDs on their lives.

# What Are Sexually Transmitted Diseases?

66 **STDs pose a serious and ongoing threat to millions of Americans. Young women, racial and ethnic populations, and men who have sex with men are particularly hard-hit by these diseases.** 99

—John M. Douglas Jr., quoted in Medline Plus, "U.S. Chlamydia Infections Hit All-Time High," November 13, 2007. www.nlm.nih.gov.

Douglas is the director of the Division of Sexually Transmitted Disease Prevention at the Centers for Disease Control's National Center for HIV/AIDS, Viral Hepatitis, STD, and TB Prevention.

66 **STDs spread through the most intimate of acts, sexual contact. And once they infect us, many of the microbes that cause most STDs today go under cover, sometimes for years. They hide out in the genital tract, undetected by their hosts, where they can spread silently from partner to partner.** 99

—Jason Eberhart-Phillips, "The Undercover World of Sexually Transmitted Diseases," El Dorado California Public Health Services, May 9, 2007. http://co.el-dorado.ca.us.

Eberhart-Phillips is the public health officer in El Dorado, California.

* Editor's Note: While the definition of a primary source can be narrowly or broadly defined, for the purposes of Compact Research, a primary source consists of: 1) results of original research presented by an organization or researcher; 2) eyewitness accounts of events, personal experience, or work experience; 3) first-person editorials offering pundits' opinions; 4) government officials presenting political plans and/or policies; 5) representatives of organizations presenting testimony or policy.

**66** Syphilis, a sexually transmitted disease that was so rare by 1998 that federal health officials had planned to declare it eliminated by 2005, has made a troubling comeback in New York City and across the nation. **99**

—Sarah Kershaw, "Syphilis Making Comeback in U.S., to Dismay of Health Officials," *New York Times,* August 12, 2007.

Kershaw is a reporter for the *New York Times.*

---

**66** Because of the ability of the [hepatitis B] virus to exist outside in the external environment for up to seven days and it could exist in such high concentration, it is often referred to as an infection which is up to a hundred times more infectious than HIV. **99**

—Samuel So, "How Serious Is Hepatitis B?" Hepatitis B Foundation, 2006. www.hepb.org.

So is the director of the Asian Liver Center and Liver Cancer Program at Stanford University, Stanford, California.

---

**66** [Chlamydia] is so common that by age 30, half of sexually active women have evidence of having had the disease at some point in their lives. The culprit is *Chlamydia trachomatis*, a bacterium transmitted during vaginal, anal, or oral sex. **99**

—Nicholas Bakalar, *Where the Germs Are: A Scientific Safari.* Hoboken, NJ: John Wiley & Sons, 2003.

Bakalar is the author of several books about various health topics.

---

66 Spreading faster than the Black Death (which took more than three centuries to kill 137 million people) and more deadly than the influenza pandemic of 1918 (which killed more people than World War I, between 20 and 40 million) AIDS is the fastest-growing and most extensive plague in human history. 99

—Monica Sweeney, *Condom Sense: A Guide to Sexual Survival in the New Millennium.* Herndon, VA: Lantern, 2005.

Sweeney is a doctor and member of the President's Advisory Council on HIV/AIDS.

66 Direct transfer of infected blood is the most efficient way to transmit HIV, but it is not the most common way. Most commonly we share HIV with one another during sexual intercourse. 99

—Gerald N. Callahan, *Infection: The Uninvited Universe.* New York: St. Martin's, 2006.

Callahan is a microbiologist and pathologist.

66 You may pass [an STD] to your baby before, during, or after the baby's birth. 99

—CDC, "STDs and Pregnancy," February 6, 2008. www.cdc.gov.

The CDC is recognized as the lead federal agency for protecting the health and safety of people at home and abroad.

**66** 'My nieta, my granddaughter, these pills are for HIV/
AIDS,' she said. 'You were infected with HIV when you
were born. You got it from your mama.' **99**

—Ana's grandmother, quoted in Jenna Bush, *Ana's Story: A Journey of Hope.* New York: HarperCollins, 2007.

Ana, who lives in a Latin American country, discovered she had HIV when she
was 10 years old.

**66** Women's economic vulnerability and dependence on
men increases their vulnerability to HIV by constrain-
ing their ability to negotiate the use of a condom, discuss fidelity with their partners, or leave risky relationships. **99**

—Geeta Rao Gupta, "How Men's Power over Women Fuels the HIV Epidemic," *BMJ*, January 26, 2002. www.bmj.com.

Gupta is the president of the International Center for Research on Women, an
organization that seeks to promote a world free of poverty in which women and
girls have opportunities equal to those of men and boys.

**66** [Adolescent] sexual relations tend to be unplanned
and sporadic, and in many cases result from pressure
or force or take place in exchange for acceptance or
financial gain. **99**

—World Health Organization, *Global Strategy for the Prevention and Control of
Sexually Transmitted Infections: 2006–2015,* May 27, 2006.

The World Health Organization directs public health for the United Nations.

# Facts and Illustrations

## What Are Sexually Transmitted Diseases?

- In 2006 the World Health Organization (WHO) reported that an estimated **340 million** new cases of curable sexually transmitted infections, such as syphilis and chlamydia, occurred worldwide in men and women aged 15 to 49 years.

- Trichomoniasis is the most common nonviral STD in the world. According to WHO, an estimated **7.4 million** trichomoniasis cases occur each year in the United States, with over **180 million** cases reported worldwide.

- According to UNAIDS, **6,800 new HIV infections** occurred each day in 2007, and **96 percent** of these were in low- and middle-income countries.

- A pregnant woman who is infected with syphilis and does not get treated has a **50 percent** chance of passing the disease to her unborn child.

- According to WHO, every year in sub-Saharan Africa **2 million** pregnant women are infected with syphilis. WHO estimates that **80 percent** of these women remain undiagnosed and do not get treated during pregnancy.

- According to the CDC, the chance of an unborn child contracting HIV from an infected mother during pregnancy is **25 percent**.

- Xiang-Sheng Chen of China's National Center for STD Control found that the total incidence of **syphilis in China increased** from 0.17 cases per 100,000 people per year in 1993 to 5.13 cases per 100,000 people per year in 2005.

- A CDC study published in 2007 states that approximately **one in four** women in the United States have HPV.

# Typical Symptoms of Common STDs

When a person is first infected with an STD, he or she may exhibit initial symptoms. A person who thinks they have been exposed to an STD and exhibits symptoms should get tested by a doctor.

| STD | Symptoms |
| --- | --- |
| **Hepatitis B** | Fatigue; nausea; fever |
| **Chlamydia** | Painful urination; lower abdominal pain |
| **Syphilis** | Painless sore where infection entered body; enlarged lymph nodes |
| **Genital Herpes** | Red bumps, blisters or sores in genital or anal areas; itching or pain in genital or anal areas |
| **Gonorrhea** | Discharge from penis or vagina; painful urination |
| **HIV** | Fever; headache; fatigue |
| **HPV** | Genital warts |
| **Trichomoniasis** | Discharge from vagina or penis; pain during urination or sex |

Sources: Mayo Clinic, "STD Symptoms: 7 STDs and Common Symptoms," February 8, 2008; Avert, "Sexually Transmitted Diseases and STD Symptoms," May 19, 2008. www.avert.org.

# Number of Chlamydia Cases Rising

The three major bacterial STDs are increasing in the United States. The following chart provides the number of cases of syphilis, chlamydia, and gonorrhea reported by state health departments from 1996 to 2006. During that period the number of chlamydia infections doubled.

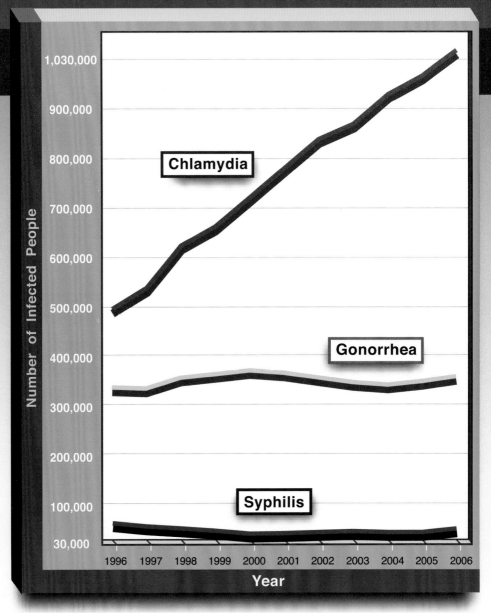

Source: Avert, "STD Statistics for USA," 2006. www.avert.org.

- According to the CDC, in 2006, **15- to 19-year-old women had the highest rate of gonorrhea** (647.9 per 100,000 population) compared to any other age/sex group.

- By age 25 **50 percent** of all sexually active young people get an STD, according to the American Social Health Association.

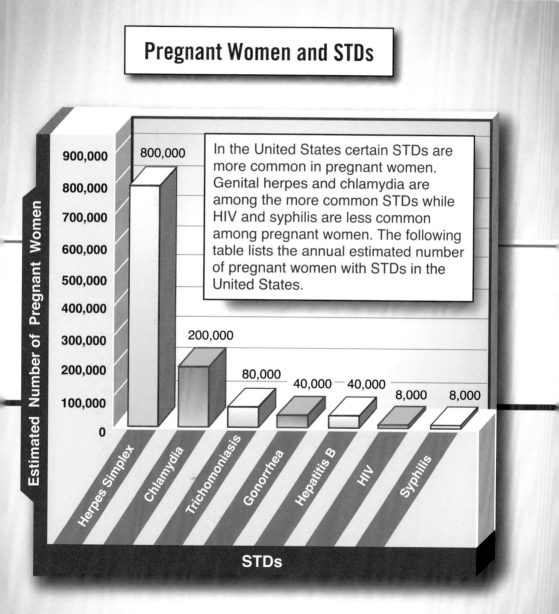

## Pregnant Women and STDs

In the United States certain STDs are more common in pregnant women. Genital herpes and chlamydia are among the more common STDs while HIV and syphilis are less common among pregnant women. The following table lists the annual estimated number of pregnant women with STDs in the United States.

Estimated Number of Pregnant Women

- Herpes Simplex: 800,000
- Chlamydia: 200,000
- Trichomoniasis: 80,000
- Gonorrhea: 40,000
- Hepatitis B: 40,000
- HIV: 8,000
- Syphilis: 8,000

STDs

Source: CDC, "STDs and Pregnancy," December 2007. www.cdc.gov.

# How HIV Replicates in the Body

Once inside the body, the HIV particle encounters CD4 cells. The HIV particle enters the body's cell. Inside the cell, HIV reverse transcriptase converts viral RNA into DNA, which is what carries the cell's genes. The newly made HIV DNA goes into the cell's nucleus and becomes a part of the cell's DNA. After copies are made, newly made HIV gather together inside the cell. This makes an immature viral particle that buds off from the cell. Next, long chains of proteins and enzymes that make up the immature viral core are cut into smaller pieces; at this time the virus becomes infectious.

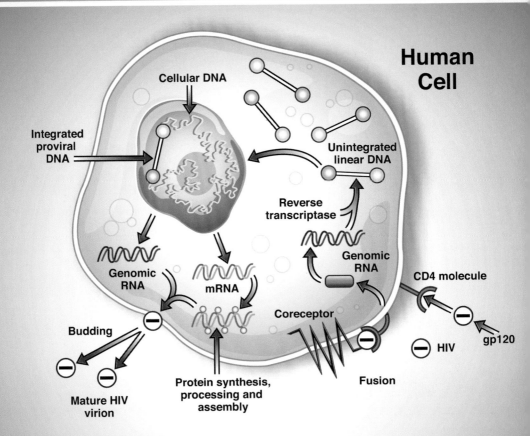

Source: National Institute of Allergy and Infectious Diseases, "How HIV Causes AIDS," November 2004. www.niaid.gov.

# STDs on the Rise Among American Teen Girls

Approximately one in four (26 percent) of young women between the ages of 14 and 19 in the United States is infected with at least one of the most common sexually transmitted diseases: human papillomavirus (HPV), chlamydia, herpes simplex virus, and trichomoniasis.

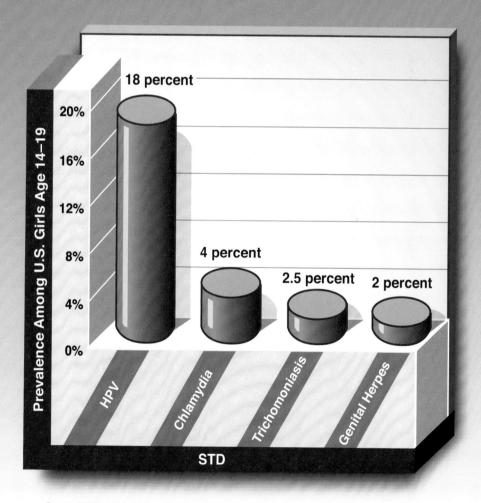

Source: MSNBC, "1 in 4 Teens Has Sexually Transmitted Disease," March 11, 2008. www.msnbc.com.

35

- A December 2005 survey published in the *Archives of Sexual Behavior* found that of the males and females ages 14 to 17 who were surveyed, **39 percent** reported having risky sex after drinking heavily, and **54 percent** reported regretting sexual activity they had engaged in after drinking.

- In 2003, according to the Henry J. Kaiser Family Foundation, **62 percent** of American twelfth graders and 33 percent of ninth graders had had sexual intercourse.

# What Are the Dangers of Sexually Transmitted Diseases?

66 My partner was diagnosed with AIDS, and I tested HIV positive. For the next basically four years we were on this roller coaster, these series of visits to the doctors, these series of moments of hell—the Kaposi's sarcoma, the Pneumocystis pneumonia, the cryptococc[al] meningitis, all of the drugs, the apparatus, the early days of AZT [zidovudine]."

—Phill Wilson, on his first years after his mid-1980s HIV diagnosis.

66 When I saw my gynecologist for a routine exam and Pap, I was diagnosed with advanced cervical cancer. Devastated by this grim prognosis, my world began to fall apart. My dream of having children instantly disappeared. To save my life, I underwent a radical hysterectomy and aggressive radiation and chemotherapy. 99

—Tamika Wilson, cervical cancer (from HPV) survivor.

STDs can affect a person in many ways, ranging from physical problems to emotional issues. Physically, how an STD affects a person depends on what type of STD he or she has contracted and at what stage the STD is diagnosed. STD effects can range from minor annoyances to fatalities.

Most initial STD symptoms are mild. Chlamydia, gonorrhea, and trichomoniasis can result in vaginal or urethral discharge, genital itching, or burning during urination. Syphilis and herpes may result in genital bumps or sores. HIV can initially be associated with a low-grade fever or rash. Genital warts may accompany a human papillomavirus infection. Hepatitis B may result in flu-like symptoms.

> **Physically, how an STD affects a person depends on what type of STD he or she has contracted and at what stage the STD is diagnosed.**

The major bacterial STDs—gonorrhea, chlamydia, and syphilis—are curable, but if they are undiagnosed, these STDs may result in severe health issues. Pelvic inflammatory disease (PID), a health issue specific to women, is one of the most severe results. Normally, a woman's cervix, the opening to the womb, prevents bacteria in the vagina from spreading up into reproductive organs. However, if the cervix is exposed to gonorrhea or chlamydia, it becomes infected. This can allow bacteria to travel up into the internal organs, making them inflamed. This may lead to PID. With PID, a woman's fallopian tubes and uterus may be damaged and result in infertility and ectopic pregnancies. In men, chlamydia and gonorrhea can cause epididymitis, a painful condition of the testicles that can result in infertility.

Syphilis can lead to severe consequences in both men and women. In the first stage of syphilis, a painless sore may develop where syphilis enters the body. If untreated, secondary syphilis will follow. Secondary syphilis results in fever, swollen lymph glands, and fatigue. In its third stage, syphilis can cause skin lesions, mental deterioration, loss of balance and vision, shooting pains in the legs, and heart disease.

The damage of bacterial STDs can be avoided if diagnosed in a timely manner, but not so with the viral STDs. These are not curable by medical means. A person who contracts genital herpes may suffer outbreaks of genital sores and blisters throughout his or her life. Ten percent of people who get infected with hepatitis B are left with a chronic infection. Chronic hepatitis B can result in severe liver disease, including cirrhosis and liver cancer. If human papillomavirus (HPV) does not clear up on its own, it can lead to cervical cancer and genital warts. A person infected with HIV must deal with it throughout his or her life. If the HIV develops into AIDS, the person is at severe risk for opportunistic infections that can lead to death.

## Can STDs Be Fatal?

Untreated HIV will lead to AIDS and ultimately death. The viral HIV DNA, which is made after HIV gets into the body, kills the body's CD4 cells, which fight diseases. If not stopped, HIV will damage enough CD4 cells so that the immune system cannot fight off infections. As a result, in 2007, according to UNAIDS, HIV/AIDS killed an estimated 2.1 million people.

Although it is the most prominent STD, HIV/AIDS is not the only STD that results in fatalities. Throughout the world, an estimated 1 million people die each year from hepatitis B and its complications of the liver. The liver is needed for several vital functions, including making clotting factors to stop bleeding from injuries and cuts, bile needed to digest food, and immune factors required to fight infections. Hepatitis B can cause cirrhosis, liver cancer, and liver failure, making it impossible for the liver to perform all of its functions.

HPV can also be fatal. According to the U.S. National Institutes of Health, 2 strains of HPV, HPV-16 and HPV-18, are responsible for about 70 percent of the cases of cervical cancer worldwide. Throughout the world, cervical cancer is estimated to cause over 233,000 deaths each year.

> With PID, a woman's fallopian tubes and uterus may be damaged and result in infertility and ectopic pregnancies.

In extreme situations, chlamydia, syphilis, and gonorrhea may also result in death. Chlamydia can cause PID, which can lead to bacteria invading and poisoning the blood. Untreated gonorrhea can also fatally poison the bloodstream. Moreover, if syphilis reaches its third stage, the syphilis bacteria may spread throughout the entire body, infecting the bones, heart, brain, and spinal cord, and result in death.

## Severe Impact on Infants

STDs are particularly dangerous to infants. If a pregnant woman is infected with an STD and does not get treatment, her newborn has a high probability of contracting the STD. Infants born with STDs are in danger of major physical damage due to their fragile immune systems.

According to the National Institute of Allergy and Infectious Diseases, untreated early syphilis in a pregnant woman results in the death of her unborn baby in up to 40 percent of cases. Children who are born with HIV are also at great risk for fatal infections. Worldwide, according to UNAIDS, 330,000 children died from HIV/AIDS in 2007.

Other STDs impacting infants are gonorrhea and chlamydia. Each can cause premature birth, eye disease, and pneumonia. Additionally, unless they are treated at birth, more than 90 percent of infants born to women with hepatitis B will carry the virus. These children are at high risk for perinatal infections and chronic liver disease as adults.

Alyson Peel, who served as a Peace Corps volunteer in Swaziland, saw firsthand the effects of STDs in children. While in Swaziland, she met a man who worked in the fields. On one visit, Peel met his youngest child, who was just two years old. "The infant was covered in scales and oozing sores such that his eyes could not open, barely recognizable as human,"[11] wrote Peel. She arranged for the father to bring the boy to a clinic for testing. The child was diagnosed with congenital syphilis. If left untreated, the child would likely have continued to suffer with neurological complications and potentially death.

## STDs Lead to Increased Risk of HIV

Even STDs that are rarely or not at all fatal can increase a person's risk of becoming infected with HIV. A person infected with an STD typically has a greater risk of acquiring HIV. This is due to the physical effects of the STDs.

> **An estimated 1 million people die each year from hepatitis B and its complications of the liver.**

A person with syphilis has an estimated 2 to 5 times increased risk of acquiring HIV infection. The genital sores from syphilis break the skin and mucous membranes, which protect the body from infections. Genital sores that come in contact with vaginal fluid, semen, or blood of an HIV-positive person make it easier for the HIV to enter the body. Other STDs that cause sores, such as herpes, cause a similar increased susceptibility to HIV.

STDs that do not result in sores, such as chlamydia, gonorrhea, and trichomoniasis, still result in a higher risk for HIV. These STDs lead to an increase of the concentration of CD4 cells, immune cells, in genital fluids. Immune cells are targets for HIV. The more immune cells in a person's genital fluids, the more likely an HIV-infected person can transmit the virus to him or her during sexual relations.

## Difficult to Diagnose

One of the major dangers of STDs is that they remain undiagnosed and untreated. Most STDs can either be cured or at least treated to lessen the damage of the STDs. However, if left undiagnosed, a person with an STD will likely suffer health problems.

> " If a pregnant woman is infected with an STD and does not get treatment, her newborn has a high probability of contracting the STD. "

The main reason people go undiagnosed is that many STDs are not accompanied by symptoms. According to the CDC, up to 75 percent of women and 50 percent of men do not experience initial symptoms from chlamydia. About 50 percent of adults with hepatitis B never experience symptoms. Some men and most women with gonorrhea exhibit no symptoms. The Mayo Clinic reports that most people with genital herpes never know they have it because the symptoms can be so mild. A person infected with HIV or HPV may not experience symptoms for years.

Because a person often will not suspect he or she has an STD, doctors recommend that all sexually active people get tested for STDs. STD tests are not a part of regular physical checkups, so a person must specifically request testing from his or her doctor.

## Encountering Prejudice

In addition to dealing with the health impacts of STDs, infected people may also have to deal with prejudice and violence. For example, in 2004 Sumitra Patel, who lived in India, discovered she had HIV. Her husband had died of AIDS in 2003. After she learned of her status, she moved to her father's house, but because of her HIV other relatives forced her to move into a hut on the outskirts of the village. Three weeks later she was found dead, lying in a pool of blood.

According to police, she was hit on the head with a sharp weapon. Patel's father blamed his nephew and brother. "A few days ago Sumitra came to visit us and she met my nephew Anil's children and interacted with them," her father said, days after the murder. "When [my brother and nephew] found out they beat her up and threatened to kill her if she was seen in the village again."[12] Patel's uncle and cousin eventually confessed to police that they killed her because she was HIV positive.

> A person with syphilis has an estimated 2 to 5 times increased risk of acquiring HIV infection.

Others with STDs do not experience violence but do experience discrimination in the way they are treated. Around the world, people have been fired from their jobs or made to leave school due to their HIV status. Other people have been asked to leave their homes or are shunned by friends and family. This discrimination is often due to both the fear people have of getting an STD and from the stigma of immoral behavior that people attach to those infected with STDs.

## Do STDs Cause Emotional Problems?

Because of the stigma and prejudice associated with STDs, studies have found that STDs adversely affect people's psychological health. Men and women with STDs, particularly those with chronic infections, often experience emotional difficulties when first diagnosed. This is partly due to the public perception that a person with an STD has done something wrong.

"I had to cope with a shattered self-perception of my sexuality," writes Curtis Finney of his genital herpes diagnosis. "I felt dirty, unlovable and untouchable."[13] According to a 2007 study in the *Herpes Monitor* of people afflicted with genital herpes, many feel like Finney. Twenty-three percent of those surveyed experienced emotional trauma due to their disease, and 37 percent stated that they thought genital herpes had ruined their lives.

These emotions can lead to depression. Studies have specifically linked HIV to an increased chance of depression. According to a 2005 report in the *Journal of Acquired Immune Deficiency Syndromes*, 22 to 45 percent of HIV-positive people develop depression. This is significantly higher than the 15 percent rate for the general population. Because of this finding, "Mental health evaluation should be an integral health care component of all HIV-infected patients receiving medical care,"[14] state the researchers of the *Journal of Acquired Immune Deficiency Syndromes* study.

## What Are the Economic Impacts of STDS?

When STDs increase to epidemic proportions in poverty-stricken countries, they not only affect the people's physical health, but also the overall economic health of the countries. These countries, already poor, do not have adequate money to devote to STD health care. As a result, infected people get sicker, spread the disease to others, and may die. This leads to a shrinking workforce for the countries. With less people to work in businesses and on farms, the countries make less money, which leads to greater poverty. Additionally, farming is neglected, leading to food shortages and countrywide malnutrition.

Many African countries are in economic crisis due to the HIV epidemic. Zambia, with one in six people infected with HIV, has experienced economic devastation due to HIV. In Zambia, where the life expectancy is below age 40, mainly due to HIV, its businesses have lost profits because they must pay the costs of absenteeism, medical care, and funerals for their HIV-stricken workers. According to the Zambia Business Coalition, 82 percent of known causes of employee deaths are HIV-related. The result is that production costs rise, and the companies make less money, bringing in less money to the country. Tied to that, people who have left the workplace due to HIV lose household income. They cannot afford to take care of their families, and the government cannot afford to take care of them.

> " Up to 75 percent of women and 50 percent of men do not experience initial symptoms from chlamydia. "

Adding to the economic problems in Zambia is loss of workers who can farm due to HIV/AIDS. AIDS is believed to have made a major contribution to the food shortages that caused a national emergency in Zambia in 2002. Unfortunately, HIV has affected several other developing countries in the same way. For this reason, international health agencies, such as WHO, stress that the world must find a way to control the epidemic of STDs like HIV/AID. Otherwise, more STD epidemics will occur throughout the world, leading already poor countries into economic crises.

# What Are the Dangers of Sexually Transmitted Diseases?

66 With no symptoms, the only way to ensure a timely diagnosis [of an STD] is screening. Otherwise, an infection can linger under the radar for many years. That is why it's not enough just to go for STD testing when you have symptoms. Every sexually active adult should consider being screened for STDs on a regular basis. 99

—Elizabeth Boskey, "How Does STD Infection Increase HIV Risk?" About.com, November, 18, 2007. http://std.about.com.

Boskey, a health education specialist, researches and writes extensively about STDs.

66 The impact of STDs is particularly severe for women. Since many STDs often cause few or no symptoms in women, they may go untreated. Women are at serious risk for complications from STDs. Some of these complications include: ectopic (tubal) pregnancy, chronic pelvic pain, infertility and cervical cancer. 99

—Cool Nurse, "STDs," 2007. www.coolnurse.com.

Cool Nurse is a Web site that was created to provide today's teens and young adults with health, fitness, and well-being information.

* Editor's Note: While the definition of a primary source can be narrowly or broadly defined, for the purposes of Compact Research, a primary source consists of: 1) results of original research presented by an organization or researcher; 2) eyewitness accounts of events, personal experience, or work experience; 3) first-person editorials offering pundits' opinions; 4) government officials presenting political plans and/or policies; 5) representatives of organizations presenting testimony or policy.

66 STDs occur worldwide, and range in severity from a nuisance to life-threatening. Some are easily cured, but others, if not treated or if incurable, can have serious effects on your health. Possible consequences include infertility, ectopic pregnancy, cirrhosis of the liver, birth defects in children and cancer. 99

—Public Health Agency of Canada, "Sexually Transmitted Diseases," January 2001. www.phac-aspc.gc.ca.

The Public Health Agency of Canada, part of the Canadian government, leads the effort to promote and protect the health of Canadians.

66 In my case, HPV is not just an STD. My mortality is attached to it. The bottom line is that I might get cancer. 99

—Dina Gruber, quoted in OnMilwaukee.com, "HPV: An STD with Life-Threatening Strings Attached," September 27, 2007. www.onmilwaukee.com.

Gruber discovered she was infected with HPV after getting an abnormal result back from her routine PAP test.

66 There is substantial biological evidence demonstrating that the presence of other STDs increases the likelihood of both transmitting and acquiring HIV. 99

—CDC, "The Role of STD Detection and Treatment in HIV Prevention," April 10, 2008. www.cdc.gov.

The CDC is recognized as the lead federal agency for protecting the health and safety of people at home and abroad.

66 Despite advances made in the treatment of HIV, liver disease from hepatitis B continues to cause serious health problems in the HIV-infected. People coinfected with both hepatitis B and HIV are 14 to 17 times more likely to die than those with hepatitis B alone. 99

—Christine Kukka, "HBV/HIV Connection: What You Need to Know," HBV Advocate, 2004. www.hbvadvocate.org.

Kukka is the U.S.-based HBV project manager for the Hepatitis C Support Project.

66 Growing up in our society, most of us come to view a sexually transmitted disease as a fate that befalls only those who have done something wrong. 99

—American Social Health Association, "Emotional Issues Overview." www.ashastd.org.

The American Social Health Association is a nonprofit organization dedicated to developing and delivering accurate, medically reliable information about STDs to the public.

66 The days that followed my herpes diagnoses were difficult, to say the least. . . . There were a million questions running through my mind: Who gave this to me? Will I ever have sex again? What did I do to deserve this? Will anyone want me when they find out? 99

—Sophia Sassoon, "Life with Herpes," June 26, 2007. www.teenwire.com.

Sassoon was diagnosed with genital herpes in her twenties.

66 [HIV]'s a bad disease, but it's a treatable disease; it's a chronic disease. People look at it the way they would look at hypertension or diabetes. You don't want it, but if you do get it, it's not the death sentence that it was 20 years ago. 99

—Harold Jaffe, quoted in The Body, "An Interview with Harold Jaffe, M.D.," February 27, 2007. www.thebodypro.com.

Jaffe is the head of the Department of Public Health at the University of Oxford in the United Kingdom.

66 My day starts very early in the morning, I get up at around about 6 o'clock to take my medication. Once I take my medication I can go back to bed and sleep off some of the side effects and be ready to get to school. I have to take nine tablets a day but some young people have to take as many as 12–14 tablets a day. 99

—Lynn, "Life Is a Struggle When You're HIV Positive," BBC News, December 1, 2005. http://news.bbc.co.uk.

Lynn is a teenager in the United Kingdom who is HIV positive.

66 It is widely known, that in the most affected countries, the [HIV/AIDS] pandemic has eroded the economic and social gains of the past thirty years. 99

—Jean-Louis Sarbib, quoted in The World Bank, "New Report Warns of Long-Term Economic Impacts from HIV/AIDS," December 1, 2004. www.worldbank.org.

Sarbib is the senior vice president of the World Bank's Human Development Network.

**"**The total estimated burden of the nine million new cases of these STDs that occurred among [American] 15- [to] 24-year-olds in 2000 was $6.5 billion (in year 2000 dollars). Viral STDs accounted for 94% of the total burden ($6.2 billion), and nonviral STDs accounted for 6% of the total burden ($0.4 billion). HIV and HPV were by far the most costly STDs in terms of total estimated direct medical costs, accounting for 90% of the total burden ($5.9 billion).**"**

—Harrell W. Chesson et al., "The Estimated Direct Medical Cost of Sexually Transmitted Diseases Among American Youth, 2000," *Perspectives on Sexual and Reproductive Health,* vol. 36, no. 1, January/February 2004. www.guttmacher.org.

Chesson, Blandford, Gift, Tau, and Irwin are economists and health researchers who worked together to determine monetary costs of STDs.

**"**Globally, all these [STD] infections constitute a huge health and economic burden, especially for developing countries where they account for 17% of economic losses caused by ill-health.**"**

—World Health Organization, *Global Strategy for the Prevention and Control of Sexually Transmitted Infections: 2006–2015.* May 27, 2006.

The World Health Organization directs public health for the United Nations.

# What Are the Dangers of Sexually Transmitted Diseases?

- Chlamydia and gonorrhea account for nearly **66 percent** of epididymitis, an inflammation of the epididymis, the tubular structure that connects the testicle with the vas deferens.

- If not adequately treated, **20** to **40 percent** of women infected with chlamydia and **10** to **40 percent** of women infected with gonorrhea may develop PID, according to the CDC's *STD Surveillance 2006* report.

- According to the CDC, approximately three to six weeks after infection with syphilis, a **chancre** (a lesion of syphilis and certain other infectious diseases, commonly an ulcer sore with a hard base) appears in the genital area where syphilis first entered the body. The chancre heals on its own within a month or two, but without treatment syphilis will enter the secondary stage.

- According to the Hepatitis B Foundation, the risk of liver cancer is **60 times greater** in those with chronic hepatitis B than those who are not infected.

- Four strains of HPV account for **80 percent** of the world's cervical cancer cases.

- The World Bank estimates that for women 15 to 44 years old in developing countries, **STDs**, not including HIV, are the **second leading cause of years of healthy life lost**, after maternal morbidity and mortality.

- Untreated AIDS leads to **death** two to five years after the first appearance of an opportunistic infection.

- According to UNAIDS, **290,000 children** died of AIDS in 2007.

- Chronic hepatitis B causes **80 percent** of the world's liver cancer. According to the World Health Organization, at least **550,000** people die each year from primary liver cancer.

- The CDC reports that untreated syphilis during pregnancy results in infant death in up to **40 percent** of the pregnancies.

- According to WHO, about **90 percent** of infants infected with hepatitis B will develop chronic hepatitis B infections.

- Without treatment, **65 percent** of newborns with herpes die.

## How Pelvic Inflammatory Disease Affects Women

Pelvic inflammatory disease (PID) results from bacteria moving up a woman's vagina, infecting her fallopian tubes, ovaries, and womb. The most common types of bacteria that cause PID are those from chlamydia and gonorrhea. Once in the reproductive organs, PID causes an infection that can lead to chronic pelvic pain, ectopic pregnancies, and infertility. An ectopic pregnancy is a complication in which the fertilized ovum is implanted outside the uterine wall, causing pain, internal and external bleeding, and sometimes death.

| Physical Damage from PID | Occurrence |
|---|---|
| Chronic Pelvic Pain | 18 percent |
| Ectopic Pregnancies | 9 percent |
| Infertility | 20 percent |

Source: Cool Nurse, "Pelvic Inflammatory Disease," 2000–2007.

## Hepatitis B and The Liver

A normal liver is soft and flexible. The liver of a person with a chronic hepatitis B infection, however, is under constant attack by the virus, which can result in the liver becoming hardened. This may cause cirrhosis, or permanent scarring of large areas of the liver. Due to the scarring, blood cannot flow through the tissue. Severe cirrhosis can lead to liver failure or liver cancer.

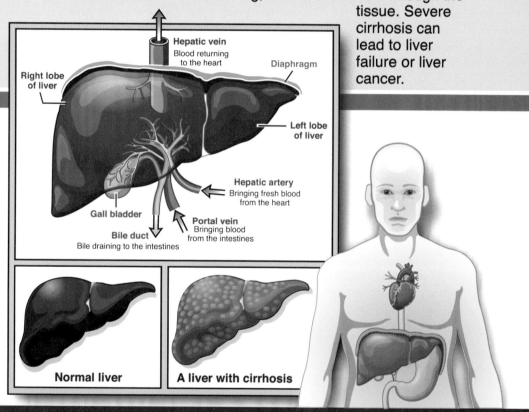

Hepatic vein
Blood returning to the heart

Diaphragm

Right lobe of liver

Left lobe of liver

Hepatic artery
Bringing fresh blood from the heart

Gall bladder

Portal vein
Bringing blood from the intestines

Bile duct
Bile draining to the intestines

Normal liver

A liver with cirrhosis

Source: Hepatitis B Foundation. www.hepb.org.

- Because people with chlamydia often do not have symptoms, the CDC estimates that approximately **2.8 million** people were newly infected with chlamydia in 2005 compared to the **976,445 new cases** that were reported.

# Common Infections Among People with HIV

Opportunistic infections are infections that do not cause disease in a person with a healthy immune system but can lead to death in a person whose immune system has been weakened by HIV. The following diagram shows the location of common opportunistic infections and what they are.

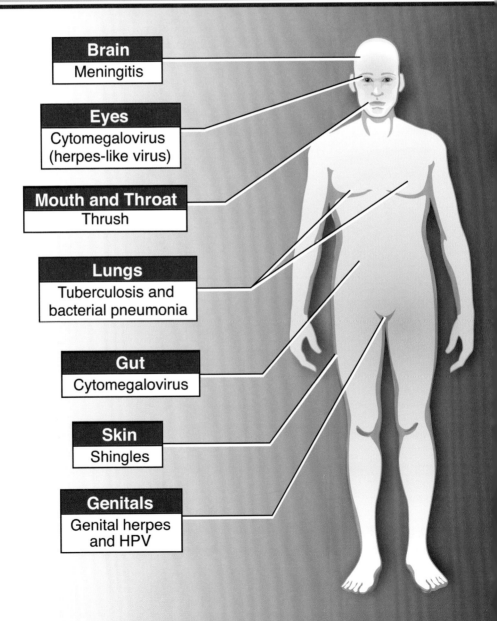

**Brain**
Meningitis

**Eyes**
Cytomegalovirus
(herpes-like virus)

**Mouth and Throat**
Thrush

**Lungs**
Tuberculosis and
bacterial pneumonia

**Gut**
Cytomegalovirus

**Skin**
Shingles

**Genitals**
Genital herpes
and HPV

Source: AIDS Education Global Information System. www.aegis.com.

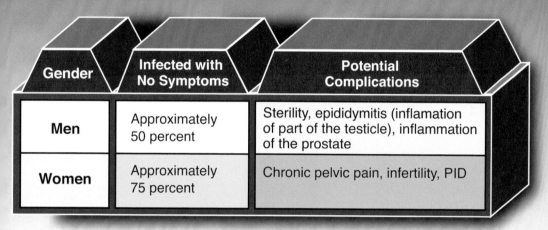

### Chlamydia Can Have No Symptoms

Chlamydia is one of the most common STDs, particularly among young people. One major problem with chlamydia is that it is often undiagnosed because people do not show symptoms. As a result, serious complications can arise.

| Gender | Infected with No Symptoms | Potential Complications |
|---|---|---|
| Men | Approximately 50 percent | Sterility, epididymitis (inflamation of part of the testicle), inflammation of the prostate |
| Women | Approximately 75 percent | Chronic pelvic pain, infertility, PID |

Source: CDC, "Chlamydia Fact Sheet," December 20, 2007. www.cdc.gov.

- In 2005 the CDC reported that in the United States direct medical costs associated with STDs were **$14.1 billion** annually.

- A person who has been infected with gonorrhea and cured is not protected from getting another infection. A new exposure to gonorrhea will cause **reinfection**, even if the person was previously treated.

- In men, prolonged infection with trichomoniasis can potentially damage their **bladders** as well as their **prostates**. In women, untreated infections can cause the **fallopian tubes** to become inflamed.

- In addition to the physical impact of genital herpes, infected people may experience **psychological impacts** including anxiety related to sexual desirability and increased depression.

# Can Changes in Behavior Prevent Sexually Transmitted Diseases?

All STDs are preventable. If people abstain from sexual relations, they reduce their chance of contracting an STD to almost zero. People who choose to engage in "safe sex" (sex with the use of condoms or sex within a monogamous relationship with an uninfected person) also significantly reduce their chance of contracting an STD.

For this reason, governments and international agencies are spending billions of dollars on prevention programs that focus on "safe sex." Developed countries, like the United States, have implemented far-reaching programs within their countries. Additionally, wealthier countries are implementing prevention programs in poorer countries that cannot afford such programs on their own.

The United States President's Plan for Emergency AIDS Relief (PEPFAR) attempts to reach people in poorer countries with high HIV prevalence rates. The PEPFAR program uses the "ABC" message. According to the PEPFAR Web site, "'A' behaviors include abstinence, including delay of sexual debut for youth; 'B' includes faithfulness to one partner or reducing the number of sexual partners; 'C' emphasizes correct and consistent condom use, where appropriate."[15]

Despites these efforts, not everyone who hears these messages practices preventive measures. For example, even with STD knowledge, many Americans practice safe sex only at the beginning of a new relationship.

"As trust develops, the likelihood of perceiving someone as having HIV goes down rapidly, and after a relatively short time," says Peter Vanable, who researches HIV/AIDS at Syracuse University. "That is not because people have gotten tests. It is because of social psychological processes, not based on knowledge about what they know about their partner, but based on personal feelings and trust."[16]

Drugs and alcohol are another factor in risky sex. People who are inebriated or high on drugs are less likely to make thoughtful sexual decisions based on their STD knowledge. According to a 2000 Kaiser Family Foundation Study, 25 percent of sexually active high school students reported using alcohol or drugs during their most recent sexual encounter.

Because of these obstacles, the United States alone sees 19 million people become infected with an STD each year. As a result, both governments and health organizations are attempting to find more innovative ways not only to get people to learn about but also to implement safe sexual behavior.

## Are Condoms Effective?

Condoms are a major part of most prevention programs. Studies have found that male latex condoms can reduce the risk for HIV, chlamydia, gonorrhea, and trichomoniasis. Additionally, condoms may reduce the transmission of HPV and genital herpes, but studies are not yet conclusive.

Condoms may be made of latex, lambskin, or polyurethane. Condoms made of latex provide the most protection against STDs. For example, according to the CDC, studies have found that with couples in which one person is infected with HIV, the regular

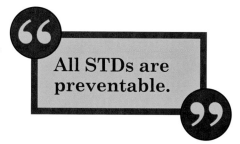

All STDs are preventable.

use of latex condoms results in the HIV-free partner having an 80 percent less chance of contracting HIV from the infected partner.

A condom works when a man wears it on his penis during sexual activity. When he ejaculates, the condom captures the man's sperm, which is where STD bacteria and viruses can live. The condom keeps the sperm from coming into contact with the genitals of his sexual partner. Additionally, the condom protects the man from coming in contact with his sexual partner's genital fluids, either sperm from another male or vaginal fluids from a female.

The Federal Drug Administration (FDA) regulates condoms in the United States. The FDA randomly tests and samples condoms to ensure their quality. According to the CDC, condom failure to prevent STDs or pregnancy is generally due to incorrect use or inconsistent use. The CDC recommends that people use a new condom with each sex act, put the condom on the penis after it is erect, and use only water-based lubricants.

## Have Safe Sex Programs Been Effective?

Uganda is an example of a country that has been able to significantly lower its HIV rates due to a combination of safe sex prevention efforts. Uganda's prevention programs focus on the ABC method. These programs are credited with helping to bring adult HIV prevalence from around 15 percent in the early 1990s to around 6.7 percent in 2005, according to UNAIDS estimates.

One of the reasons for Uganda's success is that the country's government started prevention efforts early in the HIV crisis. In 1986 President Yoweri Museveni embarked on a nationwide tour to tell people that they should abstain from sex before marriage, remain faithful to their partners, and to use condoms. Since then, Uganda's government has established agencies specifically to fight HIV.

> "Condoms made of latex provide the most protection against STDs."

With the government's support, Ugandan churches, clinics, and schools counsel people on how to prevent HIV transmission. For example, since 1987 Ugandan teachers have been trained to integrate HIV education into their school curriculum. These programs teach both abstinence and condom use as prevention methods. "While condom promotion was not a dominant element in Uganda's early response to AIDS, in more recent years, increased condom use has contributed to the continuing decline in prevalence,"[17] states Anne Peterson, global administrator for public health for USAID, an independent U.S. government agency dedicated to global health.

## Controversies with Safe Sex Campaigns

Despite their successes, safe sex programs are controversial. One of the main issues is that some people believe that advocating condom use will encourage young people to have sex.

As an alternative to "safe sex" programs, faith-based organizations have implemented "abstinence-only" programs. These programs do not provide information on condoms. Instead, they solely focus on teaching young people to abstain from sex until marriage. For example, True Love Waits is an international campaign that uses rallies, teachings through church groups, and promotional materials to encourage young people to remain sexually abstinent until marriage. From its start in 1993 to 2008, over a million young adults signed True Love Waits pledge cards stating that they would remain virgins until marriage.

> **Since 1987 Ugandan teachers have been trained to integrate HIV education into their school curriculum.**

Because of the growing popularity of abstinence-only programs, U.S. president George W. Bush asked for $191 million for abstinence education for fiscal year 2008, an increase of $28 million from fiscal year 2007. However, many disagree with this action, as recent studies have shown that abstinence-only education is not effective at preventing teenage sex.

Mathematica Policy Research Inc., on behalf of the U.S. government, recently studied the effects of abstinence-only programs. The study found that abstinence-taught teens were no more likely than other teenagers to abstain from sex or even to wait longer before losing their virginity. "Now that the government has collected its own evidence that teaching about abstinence doesn't make kids less sexually active, it's time to redirect money to comprehensive sex ed," writes Amanda Schaffer, science and medical columnist for *Slate*, an online newspaper. "The kind that teaches kids to protect themselves with condoms and is much more likely to do some good."[18]

## Testing and Partner Notification

In addition to abstinence and safe sex, another behavioral way to prevent the spread of STDs is testing and partner notification. Testing is an essential part of STD prevention because a person who knows he or she has an STD can get cured or treated. Additionally, people who know they are infected can prevent themselves from infecting others.

WHO specifically has developed the Sexually Transmitted Diseases Diagnostics Initiative, a program devoted to testing people for STDs in developing countries. Often people remain undiagnosed in developing countries because they cannot afford or do not live near health clinics that provide testing. WHO's program is devoted to finding rapid and affordable ways to diagnose STDs in these countries.

> [Abstinence-only] programs do not provide information on condoms.

Tied to testing is partner notification. Prevention programs urge people who know they are infected with an STD to let their sexual partners know. This way their partners can get tested and, if they are infected, can get treatment and not infect others. In certain states a person who has HIV is required by law to notify his or her sexual partners.

The problem with partner notification is that many people are scared to notify sexual partners of their status. They fear rejection and ridicule. "I was an irresponsible coward when I first got herpes," writes Christopher Scipio, a holistic practitioner who has and treats people with genital herpes. "Because the doctors told me that I wasn't contagious without outbreaks and because I was in the habit of using condoms, I decided that I only had to tell someone that I had herpes if and when it seemed like the relationship was turning serious and there would be regular sexual contact."[19]

To break the barriers of notifying partners, several innovative programs have been developed. In the United States, the CDC has implemented its Expedited Partner Therapy. This program intends to make notification easier on the partners of patients diagnosed with chlamydia or gonorrhea. It allows those patients to take prescriptions or medications directly to their sexual partners. This way, the partners can get appropriate treatment without having to go to their doctors for STD testing, an embarrassing ordeal for some people.

In 2005 the San Francisco Health Department implemented an Internet-based program that allows people diagnosed with a sexually transmitted disease to anonymously inform their sexual partners via e-mail. This program intends to take away the embarrassment of having to inform a partner face-to-face.

## Why Are STD Rates Rising?

Despite the many prevention programs throughout the world, STD rates continue to rise. In recent years new infections of gonorrhea, syphilis, and chlamydia have been increasing in the United States. New reports also indicate that HIV may also be on rise in the United States. For years the CDC has estimated that new infections remained around 40,000 per year. Recent studies indicate between 50,000 and 60,000 people are newly infected with HIV annually in the United States.

One of the reasons the United States is seeing a rise in rates is that people are becoming complacent in their attitude toward STDs. They see STDs as treatable diseases and not a major problem.

The CDC is seeing a rise in STDs among gay men. Men having sex with other men were initially the most at risk for HIV. The scare of contracting HIV led gay males to practice safer sex. Today some homosexual men are not as cautious in their sex lives. "I know intellectually that condomless sex is wrong, but today AIDS simply doesn't seem to be a big deal,"[20] says Roberto, a 29-year-old attorney. It is attitudes like this that public health organizations are attempting to change.

## New Prevention Initiatives

In order to fight rising STD rates, more innovative prevention programs are being tested. For example, SISTA is a peer-led program targeted at African American women. Rather than just provide information about the dangers of STDs and how to prevent them, this program seeks to raise women's self-esteem. The program leaders believe that by building women's self-esteem, women will be more likely to take charge of their sex lives by insisting on condom use or making partners wait for sex until they are in a faithful relationship.

> " In certain states [of the United States] a person who has HIV is required by law to notify his or her sexual partners. "

Innovative programs also target needle usage. Between 5 and 10 percent of HIV infections are due to injecting drug use. San Francisco's needle-exchange program allows intravenous (IV) drug users to exchange used syringes for clean, sterile ones. This and similar programs, however, are controversial because some people believe they encourage drug use.

The United States is not alone in implementing innovative prevention programs. In India the government is targeting high-risk populations. The Indian government started a pilot program that provided female condoms, (a polyurethane plastic pouch that a woman inserts into her vagina) to sex workers in an effort to reduce STDs in red light districts. The program was designed to provide 500,000 female condoms by June 2007. This effort is geared not to change behavior but to deal with the reality that risky sexual behavior will not change.

> " In recent years new infections of gonorrhea, syphilis, and chlamydia have been increasing in the United States. "

Ultimately, health care professionals believe that people must change their behaviors in order to reduce the spread of STDs. The hope is that through international efforts and innovative programs, people will not only get the prevention information, but also incorporate the recommendations into their lives.

# Can Changes in Behavior Prevent Sexually Transmitted Diseases?

66 While messages of abstinence and faithfulness are key to young and married adults, it is important to provide information on condoms to those who have sex outside or before marriage. 99

— Anne Peterson, "Testimony of Dr. Anne Peterson," USAID, May 19, 2003. www.usaid.gov.

Peterson is the USAID administrator for global health.

66 Condom possession may be a constant temptation to sin as well as an instrument of seduction. It may lead to a habit of fornication and a contraceptive mentality that may destroy a future marriage. 99

—John B. Shea, "Condom Controversy," LifeIssues.net, May 22, 2005. www.lifeissues.net.

Shea, a Catholic, is a retired physician.

Primary Source Quotes

**"For the most part kids learn about sexually transmitted diseases when they are getting diagnosed with them."**

—Julie Downs, quoted in Jonathon Potts, "Teens Are Unaware of Sexually Transmitted Diseases Until They Catch One," *Innovations Report,* April 1, 2006. www.innovations-report.com.

Downs is the lead author of a study on STDs and teenage girls and a member of the Department of Social and Decision Sciences at Carnegie Mellon.

**"We have a societal reluctance to discuss sex. And when we do talk about it, we talk about it in a moral way versus as a health issue."**

—Michael Carey, quoted in Terry Wynn, "Social Issues Linked to Rise in STDs," MSNBC, April 20, 2005. www.msnbc.msn.com.

Carey runs the Center for Health and Behavior at Syracuse University.

**"By blocking the exchange of body fluids that might contain infectious agents, latex condoms provide the best protection available against STDs."**

—Mayo Clinic, "Condoms: STD Protection Plus Effective Birth Control," May 1, 2007. www.mayoclinic.com.

The Mayo Clinic is an American not-for-profit medical practice dedicated to the diagnosis and treatment of complex illnesses.

**❝If you have the slightest, the vaguest suspicion that you might be infected, get a test. Everyone should know their HIV status.❞**

—Monica Sweeney, *Condom Sense: A Guide to Sexual Survival in the New Millennium.* Herndon, VA: Lantern, 2005.

Sweeney is a doctor and member of the President's Advisory Council on HIV/AIDS.

**❝Many of my patients have told me they do not feel safe telling their partners about their HIV status because they are afraid of being rejected.❞**

—Becky Kuhn and Eric Krock, "HIV and AIDS: Prevention for Positives,"
AIDS Videos, August 20, 2006. www.aidsvideos.org.

Kuhn is a MD from Global Lifeworks and Krock is from AIDSvideos.org.

**❝I would rather tell my partner that I am positive up front than wait for feelings to come around only to have them turned off when I say I am HIV positive.❞**

—Marvelyn Brown, "POZ Focus," *POZ,* October 2006. www.poz.com.

Brown is the ambassador and community outreach coordinator for *POZ* and *Real Health* magazines.

66 One of the most controversial issues is whether physicians may disclose the HIV status of their patients to known contacts and, further, whether failure to do so may give rise to liability if the known contact becomes HIV-positive. 99

—Laura Lin and Bryan A. Liang, "HIV and Health Law: Striking the Balance Between Legal Mandates and Medical Ethics," *Virtual Mentor,* vol. 7, no. 10, October 2005. http://virtualmentor.ama-assn.org.

Lin is a registered nurse with the California Western Health Law Society. Liang is the executive director of the Institute of Health Law Studies.

66 Why did I have unsafe sex? It felt good, I was high, I wanted guys to sleep with me. I understood the safe sex message more than most and sometimes I did use condoms, but it wasn't every time. 99

—Adam, quoted in "High-Risk Sex Lives: HIV on the Rise Again," *Independent,* November 26, 2006. www.independent.co.uk.

Adam is an HIV-positive gay man in the United Kingdom.

66 Several factors seem to contribute to this high-risk behavior, including fading memories of the early [HIV] epidemic, illicit drug use and treatment optimism. 99

—Harold Jaffe, quoted in Steve Sternberg, "HIV Infections Appear to Be Rising in the United States," *USA Today,* February 11, 2003. www.usatoday.com.

Jaffe is the head of the Department of Public Health at the University of Oxford in the United Kingdom.

❝Sexually transmitted disease is a serious health problem in America, but it is almost entirely preventable through behavior choices, especially abstinence and commitment to a mutually monogamous relationship with an uninfected partner.❞

—Tommy Thompson, quoted in Steve Sternberg, "Government Report on Condoms Stresses Abstinence," July 19, 2001. www.usatoday.com.

Thompson is the former U.S. Secretary of Health and Human Services.

❝We are going to have to continue trying to encourage people to behave in ways that prevent transmission, but always with the awareness that eradication of these diseases is little more than a hopeful fantasy, and that we will live with these microbes, for better or worse, for the rest of our lives.❞

—Nicholas Bakalar, *Where the Germs Are: A Scientific Safari.* Hoboken, NJ: John Wiley & Sons, 2003.

Bakalar is the author of several books about various health topics.

# Facts and Illustrations

## Can Changes in Behavior Prevent Sexually Transmitted Diseases?

- The U.S. President's Emergency Plan for AIDS Relief (PEPFAR), which began in 2004 and that supports community activities to prevent sexual transmission, reached nearly **61.5 million** people by September 30, 2006.

- According to the CDC, **latex condoms**, when used consistently and correctly, are **highly effective in preventing male-female sexual transmission** of HIV, the virus that causes AIDS.

- A 2006 study in the *New England Journal of Medicine* found that consistent condom use can prevent the spread of HPV in up to **70 percent** of cases.

- A National Institutes of Health study found that condom breakage and slippage occurs in an estimated **1.6 to 3.6 percent** of sexual acts, and the majority of these occurrences are due to user error.

- According to the United Nations Population Fund (UNFPA), an estimated **10.4 billion** male condoms were used worldwide in 2005.

- In the United States, 14 states require that sex education classes teach both abstinence and contraception; 19 states require **abstinence-only education**, but allow teaching contraception use; and 17 states do not give any guidance to their local school boards.

- Of 12,000 young Americans who pledged to remain virgins until marriage, **88 percent** broke their pledge, according to a study by

# Teenagers and Risky Sex

Despite several STD prevention programs throughout the United States, many sexually active teenagers engage in unsafe sex. The following table provides a breakdown, by grade and sex, of sexually active teenagers who used condoms during their last sexual encounter in the year 2005. As teens get older, their condom use declines.

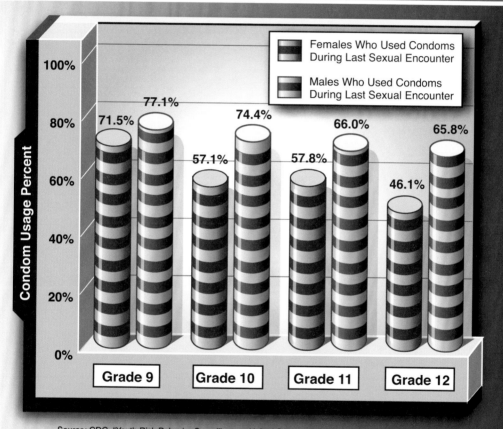

Condom Usage Percent

- Females Who Used Condoms During Last Sexual Encounter
- Males Who Used Condoms During Last Sexual Encounter

71.5% 77.1% 57.1% 74.4% 57.8% 66.0% 46.1% 65.8%

Grade 9    Grade 10    Grade 11    Grade 12

Source: CDC, "Youth Risk Behavior Surveillance—United States, 2005," June 9, 2006. www.cdc.gov.

Peter Bearman, the chair of Columbia University's Department of Sociology, and Hannah Bruckner of Yale.

- A 2004 American Social Health Association (ASHA) survey found that **93 percent** of those surveyed believe their current or most recent partner does not have an STD.

- According to the 2004 ASHA survey, about **1 out of 3** people have never discussed STDs with their sexual partner.

- Of **900,000** people living with HIV in the United States, **about one-third do not know they are infected**, according to the CDC.

# States Refusing Abstinence-Only Funding

Since 1998, the U.S. Department of Health and Human services has annually allocated $50 million in federal abstinence-only-until-marriage funding for states' use. State governments can use the funding in different sex-education areas, including school classes, community groups, state and local health departments, and media campaigns. However, the money is restricted to efforts focused on promoting abstinence-only; programs cannot promote condom use. Because of a series of reports released in 2007 that highlight the ineffectiveness of abstinence-only education programs in delaying or preventing teen sexual activity, an increasing number of states are opting out of the funding.

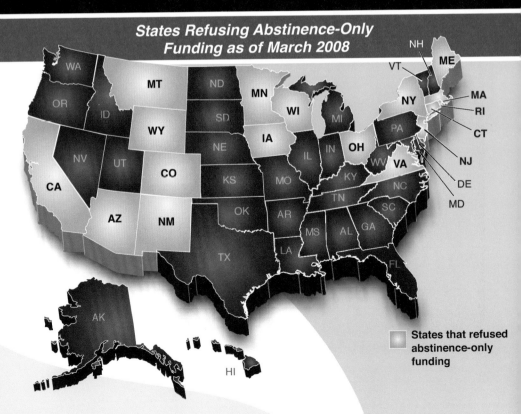

### States Refusing Abstinence-Only Funding as of March 2008

States that refused abstinence-only funding

Sources: Siecus, "Policy Updates—February 2008." February 2008. www.siecus.org; Planned Parenthood, "Governor Says No to Abstinence-Only Funds," March 7, 2008. www.plannedparenthood.org.

# Skills-Based STD Prevention Programs Are Effective

A 2005 study found that STD prevention programs that include hands-on STD risk-reduction skills may be more effective at reducing risky sexual behavior among teenagers than programs that solely provide STD information. Skills-based programs have participants engage in activities such as practicing putting condoms on anatomical models and engaging in role-playing exercises to practice condom negotiation skills. In a trial conducted in Philadelphia, participants were placed either in a skills-based STD prevention program or a control group that received general health promotion intervention. The following table shows the result, 12 months after the programs, of questionnaires and STD tests completed by 682 sexually experienced females aged 12 to 19 years who participated in the program.

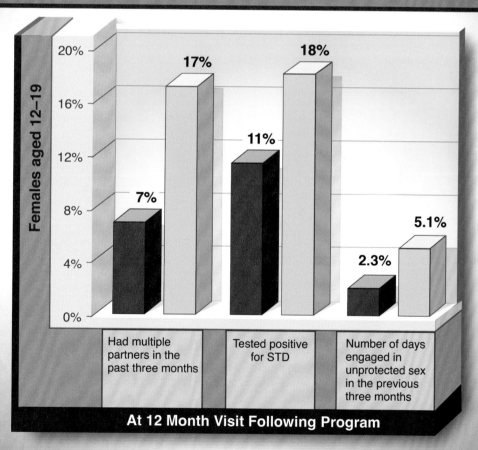

Source: "Adding a Skills-Based Component to STD Prevention Efforts May Increase Their Success Among Teenagers," *Perspectives on Sexual and Reproductive Health*, September 2005: 37 (3): 157–58 http://findarticles.com.

## Number of People Infected with HIV on the Rise in the United States

The number of people living with HIV in the United States continues to rise. Some people believe the increase in numbers is due to a growing complacency in the United States about HIV and STD risk.

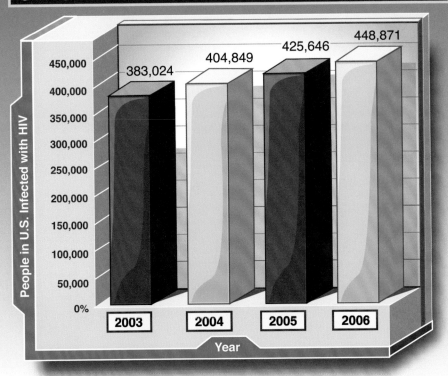

Source: CDC, "HIV Surveillance Report 2006," 2008. www.cdc.gov.

- In 2007 *POZ*, a magazine dedicated to HIV issues around the world, conducted a survey of thousands of its readers and found that **54 percent** of its HIV-positive respondents knew they were at risk for HIV before their diagnosis but did not take consistent precautions to protect themselves.

- From 2005 to 2006, according to the CDC, the U.S. chlamydia rate rose **5.6 percent**, the gonorrhea rate rose **5.5 percent**, and the syphilis rate rose **13.8 percent**.

# Can Science Eliminate Sexually Transmitted Diseases?

**When I realized I was HIV positive and pregnant, I lost all sense of hope. . . . But the medical team explained that they were going to give me medicine to save my baby. It was only after this that I started feeling happier with life, when I was told there was hope to prevent my unborn baby from getting HIV.**

—Siti, an HIV-positive Malaysian woman whose baby was born without the virus due to treatment.

Although behavioral prevention strategies have been found to reduce the spread of STDs, public health professionals believe that science is also needed to eliminate STDs. "Behavioral prevention can only achieve so much," states David Cooper, head of the National Centre in HIV Epidemiology and Clinical Research at Sydney's University of New South Wales. "Safer behaviors are not sustainable 100 percent of the time and therefore we really need to move forward on the biomedical prevention agenda."[21]

Scientists have pursued three main areas of research to reduce or eliminate STDs. These areas include STD diagnostics, STD treatment, and STD preventive measures. Scientific research has led to accurate testing methods for STDs, cures for most bacterial STDs, treatments for several viral STDs, and vaccines for hepatitis B and HPV.

## Can STDs Be Diagnosed Earlier?

The earlier an STD is detected, the better a person's chances for either recovery or relief from symptoms. Additionally, a person who knows he or she has an STD can avoid infecting others. For this reason, researchers are always looking for more accurate and quicker ways to get people diagnosed.

A recent STD testing advance was the development of an HPV test. With this test, a physician or nurse scrapes cells from a woman's cervix and puts them in a solution before the cells are examined for HPV by a lab. Studies have found this test to be more effective than a PAP smear, where cells are scraped from the cervix and placed directly on a slide to detect HPV.

> " Oraquick, an HIV test, can provide HIV test results to a person within 20 minutes of the test. "

In addition to more accurate tests, more rapid tests for STDs have become available. For example, Oraquick, an HIV test, can provide HIV test results to a person within 20 minutes of the test. Also being tested by the Federal Drug Administration are take-home HIV tests. These tests would allow people to test themselves in the privacy of their own homes.

Other rapid tests include a 30-minute chlamydia test that was approved in 2007. This test detects chlamydia on self-collected vaginal swabs, which are easier to obtain than the cervical swabs required by other tests. Syphilis can also be tested rapidly outside a laboratory with just a finger prick for a small sample of blood. Rapid tests are of great use in poverty-stricken countries where many people live far from medical facilities and cannot get there for testing and back again for results. With rapid tests, organizations like WHO can come to people using mobile medical facilities and provide immediate results.

## How Are Bacterial and Parasitic STDs Treated?

For centuries, a person who contracted syphilis was in serious trouble. Lesions, insanity, and death could result. Various treatments were tried throughout the years, but many caused even greater sickness and most did not effectively cure the disease. The discovery of penicillin in 1928 eventually led to a successful syphilis treatment. By the late 1940s penicillin became the treatment of choice for syphilis. Because of the treatment, infected people could be cured.

Over the years, medical research has led to numerous cures and treatments for bacterial and parasitic STDs. Most bacterial STDs are treated with antibiotics. Today syphilis is still typically treated with penicillin or similar antibiotics. A single dose of azithromycin or a week of doxycycline is the most common treatment for chlamydia and is successful 95 percent of the time. Treated with cephalosporin antibiotics, gonorrheal infections can be cured 95 to 99 percent of the time.

The parasitic STDs are also easily treated. Trichomoniasis can be cured with a single dose of metronidazole, a medication that kills parasites and some bacteria. Pubic lice can be treated with an over-the-counter lice-killing shampoo called a pediculicide. Because of medical research a person with pubic lice or any other bacterial or parasitic STD has a great chance of a full recovery from the disease.

## How Are Viral STDs Treated?

When HIV was first discovered, it was a death sentence. People with HIV would develop AIDS and quickly die of complications from opportunistic infections. Since then, scientists have developed several types of antiretroviral (ARV) drugs that are highly effective at fighting the HIV virus.

ARVs interfere with the HIV's ability to make DNA from RNA. ARVs are most effective when used in combination with one another. A person taking ARVs typically takes three different kinds. This combination therapy was introduced in 1996 and is known as the "triple cocktail treatment" or highly active antiretroviral therapy (HAART). Many HIV-positive people have lived for over 20 years with their disease due to HAART.

Medical research has also led to treatment of other viral STDs. Valacyclovir is an antiviral drug used to treat genital herpes. It does not cure herpes but treats the symptoms and helps keep the virus latent. Like herpes, HPV cannot be cured, but its symptoms, genital warts and precancerous cervix changes, can be treated. Treatments include cryotherapy, freezing the

> " **Medical research has led to numerous cures and treatments for bacterial and parasitic STDs.** "

abnormal cells with liquid nitrogen; conization, a biopsy that removes the abnormal areas; and loop electrosurgical excision procedure (LEEP), which removes abnormal cells with a painless electrical current. Medical science has also made advances in the treatment of chronic hepatitis B. Six FDA-approved drugs significantly decrease the risk of liver damage from the hepatitis B virus by slowing down or stopping the virus from reproducing.

## Can Mother-to-Child Transmission Be Prevented with Treatment?

Conlate Otieno, a 30-year-old HIV-infected woman in Kenya, had little hope of having healthy children. After losing her infant to AIDS in 2004 and learning she was HIV positive, Otieno feared not that she would die, but that she would never raise children. The government provided Otieno with ARV treatment. After getting on the drugs, she and her husband, who is also HIV positive, had two more children. Both children were born HIV negative. "The drugs restored my hope," said Otieno. "And I don't worry that I won't be around to take care of her,"[22] Otieno said as she held her 4-month-old baby, Josephine.

If they take ARVs, HIV-infected pregnant women can reduce their chance of passing HIV to their children from over 25 percent to just 2 percent. Additionally, scientific research has found that if an HIV-infected pregnant woman has a cesarean section versus a vaginal birth, there is a less chance that her HIV-infected blood will infect her baby.

> **Many HIV-positive people have lived for over 20 years with their disease due to HAART.**

With medical intervention, pregnant women infected with other STDs can also significantly reduce the chance of passing on the infection to their unborn children. According to the CDC, a pregnant woman with chlamydia can take erythromycin base or amoxicillin to clear her infection before childbirth, which is when a baby can get infected with chlamydia. Like chlamydia, herpes can be passed to the baby during birth, but doctors have found that women with active herpes lesions at time of delivery can prevent transmission to their baby by having a cesarean section. Gonorrhea also may infect a baby during birth, resulting in blindness. To combat this, in the United States all babies are given medicines when born to help prevent this.

Because syphilis can pass to the infant during pregnancy, the CDC recommends infected pregnant women take penicillin to reduce transmission chances. Hepatitis B can also pass to an unborn baby during pregnancy. If a pregnant woman has hepatitis B, the Hepatitis B Foundation recommends that the newborn receive the hepatitis B vaccine within the first 12 hours of his or her life to protect the baby from a chronic infection. Because of advances in scientific prevention of mother-to-child transmission, millions of children have been saved from major health issues.

## Problems with STD Treatment

Despite the advances in STD treatments, medical researchers must contend with treatment-related issues. Certain STDs can mutate and become resistant to treatment. For example, HIV is constantly mutating, and treatment may eventually become ineffective. Cleve Jones, who has been HIV positive for over 20 years, has switched ARV combinations many times due to his body developing resistance to the drugs. "My experience has been that with each combination that I've used, I've been able to get about two, two and a half, three years out of that combination,"[23] explains Jones.

> " If they take ARVs, HIV-infected pregnant women can reduce their chance of passing HIV to their children from over 25 percent to just 2 percent. "

Gonorrhea also has mutated over the years. According to the CDC, resistance to fluoroquinolones, antibiotics used to treat gonorrhea since 1993, increased among heterosexuals from 0.6 percent in 2001 to 6.7 percent in 2006. Prior to that, gonorrhea had become resistant to penicillin.

Medical researchers are working to stay a step ahead of these problems by discovering new ways to fight the diseases. For years four classes of HIV medications existed. Each worked somewhat differently to stop HIV from multiplying. In 2007 the FDA approved Isentress, the first drug of a new class of ARVs. Isentress is an integrase inhibitor that blocks integration of HIV into a cell.

Researchers are also keeping pace with gonorrhea mutations. Cephalosporins are a new type of drug to fight gonorrhea. As of 2008 no cases of gonorrhea were resistant to these antibiotics. Scientists plan to continue to work to find drugs to fight any further mutations of gonorrhea or any other STD.

# Finding Scientific Ways to Prevent STDs

Medical researchers not only search for ways to treat and cure STDs but also how to medically prevent STDs. One area under current research is microbicides. A microbicide is any cream, gel, or foam that can be applied to the vagina or rectum and that can kill disease-causing organisms such as STD viruses or bacteria.

> "A microbicide is any cream, gel, or foam that can be applied to the vagina or rectum and that can kill disease-causing organisms such as STD viruses or bacteria.

Microbicides are in the research stage, but if developed could be a major way to prevent STDs. "Topical microbicides just makes it a lot easier for women. It gives them a degree of control,"[24] said Anthony Fauci, director of the National Institute of Allergy and Infectious Diseases at the National Institutes of Health. According to the Global Microbicide Campaign, as of February 2008, 13 microbicide candidates were in clinical development.

Vaccines are substances that introduce a whole or partial version of a microorganism into the body in order to train a body's immune system to defend itself if that organism threatens to cause an infection. Currently people can get vaccinated against two major STDs—hepatitis B and the sexually transmitted strains of HPV.

In 1982 Merck & Co., a leading drug company, came out with a hepatitis B vaccine. Between 1982 and 2002, 40 million infants and children and 30 million adults received the hepatitis vaccine. In 2002 the CDC estimated that only 79,000 new hepatitis B infections occurred versus between 200,000 and 300,000 in 1982.

The most recently approved STD vaccine is the HPV vaccine, which protects the body from HPV types 6, 11, 16, and 18. After testing 11,000 women around the world with no adverse side effects, the FDA approved the vaccine in 2007. The CDC recommends that females should get the vaccine before they are sexually active. Studies have found the vaccine is nearly 100 percent effective in preventing diseases caused by the four HPV types.

Other vaccines for STDs are currently under research. In 2008 the Herpevac Trial for Women is testing a herpes vaccine in women. Scientists have also been actively searching for an HIV vaccine since the virus was first identified. Unfortunately, in 2007 the most promising vaccine prospect suffered a major setback. Merck & Co. spent a decade developing an HIV vaccine, and it failed. However, research for an HIV vaccine continues with major funding from organizations such as the Bill and Melinda Gates Foundation.

## Controversies with Vaccines

Although vaccines are considered by many the best way to eliminate diseases, they are not without controversy. One controversial issue is whether governments should require STD vaccines. Vaccines for STDs concern people because of the potential harmful effects of the vaccines. Additionally, some believe that requiring children to get vaccines that prevent sexually transmitted diseases gives the message that premarital sex is acceptable.

Once the HPV vaccine came out, 16 U.S. states began the process to require middle school girls to get this vaccine prior to registering for school. Many people have protested making the vaccine mandatory. One concern is that the vaccine has not been in use long enough to know if it could cause harmful side effects. Another concern of parents is the moral implications. "Giving the HPV vaccine to young women could be potentially harmful," states Bridget Maher of the Family Research Council, a U.S. organization whose mission is to uphold conservative marriage and family values, "because they may see it as a license to engage in premarital sex."[25]

The hepatitis B vaccine initially met with some similar arguments against mandatory vaccination. However, because of its success at reducing hepatitis B infections, U.S. states began enacting laws requiring the vaccine. Today all but three states require hepatitis B as a childhood vaccination.

> **Today all but three states require hepatitis B as a childhood vaccination.**

Despite all the controversies and concerns, health care professionals and researchers believe that vaccines are the best way to significantly reduce and potentially eradicate STDs. "We don't vaccinate just to protect our children. We also vaccinate to protect our grandchildren and their grandchildren," states the CDC. "With one disease, smallpox, we 'stopped the leak' in the boat by eradicating the disease. Our children don't have to get smallpox shots any more because the disease no longer exists."[26] Health care professionals look toward a future when STD vaccines result in similar success.

# Can Science Eliminate Sexually Transmitted Diseases?

> **❝Some social conservatives continue to fight [Virginia's bill that would require middle school girls to get the HPV vaccine], out of fear the new law will encourage youth to be sexually active.❞**

—The *Virginian-Pilot* editors, "Back to Square One on HPV Vaccine," *Virginian-Pilot*, January 17, 2008.

The *Virginian-Pilot* serves more than 600,000 residents in southeastern Virginia and northeastern North Carolina.

> **❝If you really want to have cervical cancer rates fall as much as possible as quickly as possible, then you want as many people to get vaccinated as possible.❞**

—Mark Feinberg, quoted in Rob Stein, "Cervical Cancer Vaccine Gets Injected with a Social Issue," *Washington Post*, May 30, 2005. www.washingtonpost.com.

Feinberg is the vice president of medical affairs and policy of Merck, the company that produces the HPV vaccine Gardasil.

Bracketed quotes indicate conflicting positions.

* Editor's Note: While the definition of a primary source can be narrowly or broadly defined, for the purposes of Compact Research, a primary source consists of: 1) results of original research presented by an organization or researcher; 2) eyewitness accounts of events, personal experience, or work experience; 3) first-person editorials offering pundits' opinions; 4) government officials presenting political plans and/or policies; 5) representatives of organizations presenting testimony or policy.

66 **Some thirty years after the beginning of the pandemic, there is still no vaccine against HIV. And isn't clear that there ever will be.** 99

—Gerald Callahan, *Infection: The Uninvited Universe.* New York: St. Martin's, 2006.

Callahan is a microbiologist and pathologist.

66 **Development of vaccines is particularly important for STDs, since change in sexual behavior is so difficult to accomplish and document.** 99

—Myron S. Cohen and Joseph J. Eron, "Biological HIV Prevention Strategies: Reducing Infectiousness, Susceptibility, and the Efficiency of Transmission," Medscape, June 27, 2001. www.medscape.com.

Cohen and Eron are medical doctors who research HIV and prevention methods.

66 **If immediate syphilis testing were provided as part of HIV-testing programs for all pregnant women in Haiti who currently have access to prenatal care, over 1,000 cases would be avoided each year, along with over 1,000 stillbirths and neonatal deaths.** 99

—Daniel W. Fitzgerald, quoted in Weill Cornell Medical College, "Rapid Syphilis Testing in Haiti Will Prevent Congenital Disease and Stillbirths," May 28, 2007. http://news.med.cornell.edu.

Fitzgerald is an assistant professor of medicine at Weill Cornell Medical College.

66 **[ARVs] bring people back from the brink of death. They bring people who are desperately sick back into productivity, into activity. They call it, 'the Lazarus Effect.'** 99

—Stephen Lewis, quoted in CTV.ca, "Drug Cost Key to Africa's AIDS Fight: UN's Lewis," July 31, 2004. www.ctv.ca.

Lewis is the Canadian representative on AIDS for the United Nations.

66 **I tell you, it's funny because the only time I think about HIV is when I have to take my medicine twice a day.** 99

—Magic Johnson, "Magic Johnson Pushes HIV Awareness," CNN, November 24, 2004. www.cnn.com.

Johnson, former famous NBA player, was diagnosed with HIV in 1991 and has since become a prominent HIV awareness advocate.

66 **Only a decade ago there were no treatment options. Although there is still no complete cure for hepatitis B, there are 6 approved drugs for adults (2 for children) and many promising new drugs in development.** 99

—The Hepatitis B Foundation, "Approved Drugs for Adults," 2006. www.hepb.org.

The Hepatitis B Foundation is a nonprofit organization dedicated to the global problem of hepatitis B. The Foundation supports research, promotes disease awareness, and supports immunization and treatment initiatives.

**"As a user-controlled technology, microbicides would fill an important prevention gap for women and men who are unable to successfully negotiate mutual monogamy or male condom use."**

—Global Campaign for Microbicides, "The Need." www.global-campaign.org.

The Global Campaign for Microbicides is an international effort to build support among policy makers, opinion leaders, and the general public for increased investment in microbicides.

**"I also feel so fortunate that Dr. Bowers gave me the HPV test. Without that, I probably wouldn't have found out about my [pre-cancerous cells in the cervix] until cancer had already developed."**

—Jodi McKinney, "The HPV Test: Real-Life Results," Digene HPV Test, 2008. www.thehpvtest.com.

McKinney had normal PAP results for years and, after her doctor recommended an HPV test in addition to her PAP smear, discovered she had precancerous HPV cells.

**"Changing behavior . . . could achieve limited degree of success . . . but it isn't going to completely stop the [AIDS] epidemic, whereas if we could truly come up with a highly protective vaccine, we could achieve that goal in the long run."**

—David Ho, quoted in PBS, "Interview with David Ho," *Frontline*, May 30, 2006. www.pbs.org.

Ho was named *Time*'s 1996 Man of the Year for his work in the development of the triple cocktail treatment for HIV-infected people.

**❝Even where prevention scores victories, as in Uganda, the [HIV] epidemic continues, and the question of treatment for infected people demands to be addressed.❞**

—Alexander Irwin, Joyce Millen, and Dorothy Fallows, "Myth Four: Prevention Versus Treatment," The Body, April 2003. www.thebody.com.

Irwin, Millen, and Fallows are authors of *Global AIDS: Myths and Facts.*

---

**❝The advantage of point of care [STD] tests is that they can enable treatment to be given on the spot, rather than hoping that the patient will return for treatment.❞**

—WHO, "Sexually Transmitted Infections," 2001. www.who.int.

The World Health Organization directs public health for the United Nations.

---

# Facts and Illustrations

## Can Science Eliminate Sexually Transmitted Diseases?

- In a study at McGill University in Montreal, the HPV test correctly spotted **95 percent** of cervical cancers while the PAP test found **55 percent**.

- According to the World Health Organization (WHO), more than **20 rapid syphilis tests** are commercially available.

- The Brazilian government plans to increase the number of pregnant women tested for HIV and syphilis from 1.4 million to **2.3 million** and from 2.1 million to **4.8 million**, respectively, by 2011.

- According to Avert, an international AIDS charity organization, as of December 2006 an estimated **7.1 million** of the people living with HIV in low- and middle-income countries urgently needed ARV medication, but only 2.015 million had access to the drugs.

- Selzentry, an ARV that fights HIV, was approved by the FDA in 2007 and costs **$10,600 per year**.

- In Kenya, the United States President's Emergency Plan for AIDS Relief (PEPFAR) funds more than **70 percent** of the nation's supply of AIDS drugs, which are distributed at no charge, according to the Kenya National AIDS Council.

- In 2008 two FDA-approved treatment options were available in the United States for children with **chronic hepatitis B**.

- Valacyclovir, an antiviral drug that fights genital herpes, has been found to reduce the risk of spreading genital herpes to an uninfected sex partner by **48 percent**.

- PEPFAR supported approximately **4,863 service outlets** for prevention of mother-to-child HIV transmission by September 30, 2006.

- By 2004, global investors had given **$142 million** toward microbicide research.

# Distance to Health Care Facilities a Problem in Poor Countries

The reason many people in developing countries are not diagnosed with STDs is that they live too far from medical facilities. Because they usually lack modern transportation, it is difficult for them to get to the facility, test for STDs, then return later for results. The following chart shows the average distance to the nearest health care facility for the poorest fifth of the population.

| Country | Average Distance to a Health Care Facility (km) |
|---|---|
| Niger | 26.9 |
| Chad | 22.9 |
| Madagascar | 15.5 |
| Bolivia | 11.8 |
| Haiti | 8.0 |
| Benin | 7.5 |
| Zimbabwe | 6.8 |
| Tanzania | 4.7 |
| Uganda | 4.7 |

Source: WHO. www.who.int.

## Rapid Syphilis Tests

Health agencies are using point of care (rapid) syphilis tests as a way to test people in developing countries who cannot get to medical centers. Rapid syphilis tests can be either treponemal or nontreponemal. A nontreponemal test is specific and can distinguish between a present or inactive case infection. A treponemal test does not distinguish between the two. Both types of tests provide results within 30 minutes, but the pros and cons of each type must be weighed when determining what type to use. The following chart lists the pros and cons of each type of test.

| Test Type | Pros | Cons |
|---|---|---|
| **Nontreponemal** | Simple to perform | Requires electricity for refrigerator and rotator needed for testing |
| | Can distinguish between active and past infection | Cannot be used with whole blood |
| | | False negative tests can occur |
| **Treponemal** | Simple to perform | Cannot distinguish between active and past infection |
| | Can be used with whole blood, serum, or plasma | |
| | Can be transported and stored at temperatures below 30 degrees Celsius | |

Source: WHO.www.who.int.

- According to WHO, the hepatitis B vaccine is **95 percent** effective in preventing chronic infections from developing.

- The three-shot hepatitis B vaccine series for children in the United States usually costs **$75 to $165**.

# HPV Vaccine's Potential to Prevent Cervical Cancer

In 2008, it is estimated that 11,070 women in the United States will get cervical cancer. In 2006, the FDA approved Gardasil, a vaccine to prevent people from getting infection from human papillomavirus (HPV) types 6, 11, 16, and 18. HPV types 16 (HPV-16) and 18 (HPV-18) cause approximately 70 percent of cervical cancers while HPV types 6 and 11 cause 90 percent of genital warts worldwide. Clinical trials found Gardasil to be between 95 and 100 percent effective at preventing these four types of HPV.

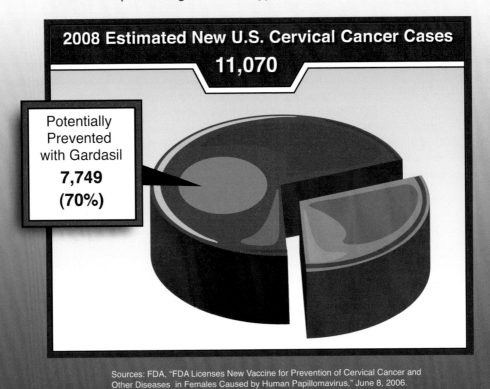

**2008 Estimated New U.S. Cervical Cancer Cases**
**11,070**

Potentially Prevented with Gardasil
**7,749**
**(70%)**

Sources: FDA, "FDA Licenses New Vaccine for Prevention of Cervical Cancer and Other Diseases in Females Caused by Human Papillomavirus," June 8, 2006. www.fda.gov; National Cancer Institute, 2008. "Cervical Cancer," www.cancer.gov.

- Both the hepatitis B vaccine and HPV vaccine are **recombinant vaccines**, which mean they **do not contain any live biological product** or DNA.

- In 2006 the FDA reported that studies of 21,000 women who received Gardasil, an HPV vaccine, showed that in women who had not already been infected, Gardasil was nearly **100 percent** effective in preventing precancerous cervical lesions, precancerous vaginal and vulvar lesions, and genital warts caused by infection of the four types of HPV the vaccine protects against.

## U.S. Cases of Cipro-Resistant Gonorrhea on the Rise in Men

For years, doctors treated gonorrhea with Cipro, a strong antibiotic; however, in recent years, gonorrhea has become resistant to this drug. In 2005 the CDC discovered that nearly 7 percent of gonorrhea cases among heterosexual men in a 2004 survey of 26 U.S. cities were drug-resistant to Cipro. In 2001 only about 0.6 percent of gonorrhea cases among heterosexual men were drug resistant. The rise in resistance requires medical researchers to develop new antibiotics that can fight the mutated gonorrhea bacteria.

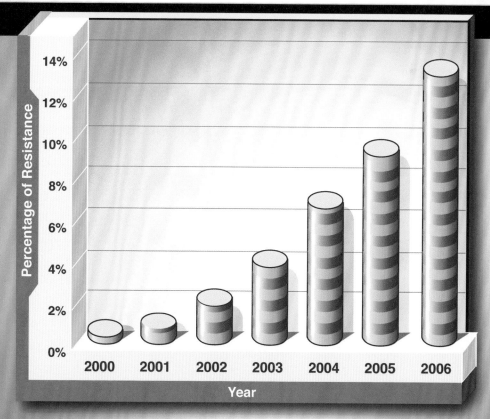

Source: CDC, 2006. www.msnbc.msn.com.

## Only Six States Do Not Require Hepatitis B Vaccinations

Forty-four states require elementary school students to have hepatitis B vaccinations. The states that do not require vaccinations for entry into elementary school are West Virginia, Vermont, South Dakota, Montana, Maine, and Alabama.

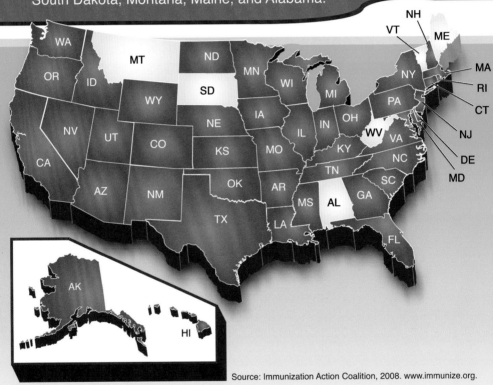

Source: Immunization Action Coalition, 2008. www.immunize.org.

# Key People and Advocacy Groups

**American Sexually Transmitted Disease Association:** ASTDA is an American organization devoted to the control and study of sexually transmitted diseases. It does so by supporting medical, epidemiologic, laboratory, social, and behavioral STD studies and research; recognizing outstanding contributions in STD control with the organization's awards; and providing information concerning STDs through its ASTDA *Sexually Transmitted Diseases* journal that publishes peer-reviewed articles on STD research and studies. In 2008 the organization cosponsored the CDC's biannual Sexually Transmitted Diseases Conference.

**American Social Health Association:** This U.S. nonprofit organization was established in 1914 and is the country's leading authority on sexually transmitted disease information. Through brochures, pamphlets, books, and other public awareness methods, this organization educates the public to understand, prevent, and destigmatize sexually transmitted diseases.

**Baruch Blumberg:** Blumberg, a medical anthropologist, discovered the hepatitis B virus in 1965. He went on to develop a diagnostic test and vaccine for hepatitis B. In 1976 Blumberg won the Nobel Prize for his hepatitis B work and findings.

**George W. Bush:** Bush, the forty-third president of the United States, announced the President's Emergency Plan for AIDS Relief (PEPFAR) in his State of the Union address on January 28, 2003. PEPFAR is a five-year, $15 billion approach to combating HIV/AIDS around the world.

**Mark R. Dybul:** Dybul serves as the U.S. global AIDS coordinator. As coordinator, he leads the implementation of President Bush's Emergency Plan for AIDS Relief. Through PEPFAR, the U.S. government works with international, national, and local leaders worldwide to support HIV/AIDS prevention, care, and treatment programs.

**Robert Gallo:** In 1984 Gallo, a U.S. medical researcher at the National Cancer Institute, announced that he had isolated the virus that causes AIDS. During his research he used the virus provided by the CDC. In 1983 Luc Montagnier and his coworkers at the Pasteur Institute believed they isolated the virus that causes AIDS and sent the virus, named lymphadenopathy-associated virus (LAV), to the CDC. The CDC passed the virus to the National Cancer Institute for research. For years the Pasteur Institute and National Cancer Institute argued over who had isolated the virus and what its name should be. Eventually, in May 1986, the International Committee on the Taxonomy of Viruses ruled that the virus be named Human Immunodeficiency Virus (HIV).

**David Ho:** Ho is a physician and scientist who first theorized that combining protease inhibitor drugs with other HIV medications would provide a more effective way to treat the disease. In 1996 this led to the "cocktail treatment," or combination of HIV drugs for treatment of HIV, that has resulted in dramatic reductions in AIDS-associated mortality. Because of his work, Ho was named *Time* magazine's 1996 Man of the Year.

**Immunization Action Coalition:** This organization works to increase immunization rates and prevent disease. It does so by creating and distributing educational materials for health professionals and the public that provide information about safe and effective immunization services. One way it educates the public is through three periodicals it produces, including *Needle Tips, Vaccinate Adults,* and *Vaccinate Women,* with a combined circulation of 390,000. Additionally, within the IAC is the Hepatitis B Coalition, a program that specifically promotes hepatitis B vaccination.

**Magic Johnson:** Johnson, a retired National Basketball Association player for the Lakers, went public with his HIV diagnosis in 1991. Since then he has been an advocate for HIV/AIDS prevention. Johnson founded the Magic Johnson Foundation, which donates needed funds to organizations that provide HIV/AIDS prevention and health care education to the minority community.

**National Vaccine Information Center:** This nonprofit organization was founded in 1982 and advocates vaccine safety and informed consent in the mandatory vaccination system. NVIC cofounders worked with Congress to pass the National Childhood Vaccine Injury Act of 1986. This law created a federal vaccine injury compensation program, mandated that doctors give parents vaccine benefit and risk information, and required the recording and reporting of vaccine injuries and deaths.

**Thomas Parran:** Parran, a physician, was sworn in as the surgeon general of the United States on April 6, 1936. During his time as surgeon general he implemented a syphilis control campaign and was able to raise funds to identify and treat syphilis through the National Venereal Disease Control Act of 1938.

**Peter Piot:** Piot, who earned a medical degree from the University of Ghent and a Ph.D. in microbiology from the University of Antwerp, Belgium, became the executive director of UNAIDS when it was created in 1995. UNAIDS is the Joint United Nations Programme on HIV/AIDSUNAIDS. Under his leadership, UNAIDS has become the chief advocate for worldwide action against AIDS.

# Chronology

**1932–1972**
The U.S. Public Health Service (PHS) conducts the Tuskegee Syphilis Experiment, an experiment on 399 black men in the late stages of syphilis. These men are not told what disease they are suffering from or its seriousness. The doctors have no intention of curing them of syphilis at all.

**1494**
The first well-recorded STD outbreak of what will become known as syphilis occurs among French troops as they besiege Naples, Italy.

**1945**
Alexander Fleming, Ernst Chain, and Howard Florey share the Nobel Prize in physiology or medicine for the discovery and isolation of penicillin. Soon after, it becomes an effective way to cure both gonorrhea and syphilis.

**1984**
The retrovirus responsible for AIDS is independently discovered by Luc Montagnier of the Pasteur Institute in Paris, France, and Robert Gallo of the National Cancer Institute in Washington, D.C. It is later named HIV.

**1879**
Albert Neisser discovers *Neisseria gonorrheaoe*, the bacteria that causes gonorrhea. For years prior to the discovery, gonorrhea was often misdiagnosed as syphilis.

**1500**  **1920**  **1940**  **1960**  **1980**

**1976**
Baruch Blumberg wins the Nobel Prize in medicine for his discovery of the hepatitis B virus. In the prior decade, he and his colleagues discovered the virus, developed the blood test that is used to detect the virus, and invented the first hepatitis B vaccine.

**1906**
The first effective test for syphilis, the Wassermann test, is developed. It produces some false positive results, but overall is a major advance in the prevention of syphilis.

**1980**
*Time* magazine reports that as many of 30 percent of the U.S. population has been infected with genital herpes, a viral STD that is incurable.

**1564**
Italian physician Gabriele Falloppio authors the first known published description of condom use. He claims that during his trial of 1,100 men using a linen sheath during sex, they were protected from syphilis.

**1981**
A high prevalence of both a rare type of skin cancer, Kaposi's sarcoma, and pneumonia are found in gay men in New York and California. These are the first documented cases of AIDS.

**1986**

A hepatitis B vaccine produced by recombinant DNA technology is licensed. A recombinant vaccine is synthetically prepared and does not contain blood products.

**1997**

U.S. president William Clinton apologizes for the U.S. government's involvement in the Tuskegee Syphilis Experiment.

**2000**

According to a report by the National Institutes of Health, correct and consistent use of latex condoms reduces the risk of HIV/AIDS transmission by approximately 85 percent relative to risk when unprotected.

**1987**

AZT (zidovudine), the first antiretroviral drug, becomes available to treat HIV patients after a successful clinical trial.

**1996**

*Time* magazine names David Ho "Man of the Year" for development of the "triple cocktail method" of combining three or more antiretrovirals (ARV) to fight HIV. The drugs change AIDS from a death sentence to a manageable chronic illness.

**2007**

The U.S. Centers for Disease Control and Prevention reports that in the prior year more than 1 million chlamydia cases were reported in the United States. This is the highest number of cases reported for an STD in the country.

**1985 — 1990 — 1995 — 2000 — 2005**

**1990**

The World Health Organization founds the Sexually Transmitted Diseases Diagnostics Initiative to improve care for patients with sexually transmitted infections (STIs) in resource-limited settings through improved rapid testing and diagnostics.

**2001**

During the twentieth year of AIDS, more than 36 million people worldwide are living with the AIDS virus, with more than 16,000 people becoming newly infected each day.

**2006**

The U.S. Food and Drug Administration (FDA) announces the approval of Gardasil, the first vaccine developed to prevent cervical cancer, precancerous genital lesions, and genital warts due to human papillomavirus (HPV) types 6, 11, 16, and 18. The vaccine is approved for use in females 9 to 26 years of age.

**1994**

A study finds that if pregnant women infected with HIV take the drug AZT, they significantly reduce the rate of maternal transmission of HIV. The study reports that with AZT, chance transmission is 8 percent as opposed to 25 percent without the drug.

**2003**

In his State of the Union address, U.S. president George W. Bush asks Congress to commit $15 billion for President's Emergency Program for AIDS Relief (PEPFAR) over the next five years to fight AIDS in the nations of Africa and the Caribbean.

**2004**

The *Journal of Gastroenterology and Hepatology* publishes a study that reports on the outcome of Taiwan's mass hepatitis B vaccination program, started in 1984. The program led to a decline from 10 percent to less than 1 percent in hepatitis B carrier rates among children.

# Related Organizations

## Avert

4 Brighton Rd.

Horsham, West Sussex RH13 5BA, United Kingdom

phone: 44 (0)1403 210202

Web site: www.avert.org

Avert is an international AIDS charity with HIV and AIDS awareness projects in countries with a particularly high rate of infection, such as South Africa, or with a rapidly increasing rate of infection, such as India. Avert also provides HIV/AIDS prevention, treatment, and history information to people all over the world through its Web site.

## Global Alliance for Microbicides

1800 K St. NW

Washington, DC 20006

phone: (202) 822-0033

fax: (202) 457-1466

e-mail: info@global-campaign.org

Web site: www.global-campaign.org

The Global Campaign for Microbicides is an international effort to increase investment in research into microbicides and other user-controlled prevention methods for STDs. The alliance is dedicated to raising awareness and political support for increased funding for microbicide research, female condom, and cervical barrier methods. On its Web site is the latest news in microbicide research and clinical trials.

## Hepatitis B Foundation

3805 Old Easton Rd.

Doylestown, PA 18902

phone: (215) 489-4900

fax (215) 489-4913

e-mail: info@hepb.org

Web site: www.hepb.org

The Hepatitis B Foundation is the only U.S. national nonprofit organization solely dedicated to the global problem of hepatitis B. The foundation funds research; promotes disease awareness; supports immunization
and treatment initiatives; and serves as a main source of information for
patients, the medical and scientific community, and the general public. Its
Web site includes the latest information about treatments, clinical trials,
and statistics concerning hepatitis B.

## National Institutes of Health

9000 Rockville Pike

Bethesda, MD 20892

phone: (301) 496-4000

e-mail: NIHinfo@od.nih.gov

Web site: www.nih.gov

The National Institutes of Health funds medical research for the U.S.
government. Its Web site provides information on several clinical trials regarding treatments and vaccines for STDs. The Web site's Sexually Transmitted Diseases Page provides information about treatment, prevention,
and medical facts of the major STDs.

## Planned Parenthood Federation of America

434 W. 33rd St.

New York, NY 10001

phone: (212) 541-7800

fax: (212) 245-1845

Web site: www.plannedparenthood.org

With 107 locally governed affiliates nationwide and more than 860
health centers, Planned Parenthood is a health care provider and educator

dedicated to women's health issues. One of its missions is to reduce the spread of sexually transmitted infections through testing and treatment. Its Web site provides specific information about STDs, their causes, treatments, and prevention methods.

### United Nations Children's Fund (UNICEF)

3 United Nations Plaza

New York, NY 10017

phone: (212) 326-7000

fax: (212) 887-7465

Web site: www.unicef.org

UNICEF is a part of the United Nations with the mission to overcome poverty, violence, disease, and discrimination for children throughout the world. UNICEF works in 191 countries through its country programmes and national committees. UNICEF works to prevent mother-to-child prevention of HIV/AIDS, provide treatment for HIV/AIDS to children, and prevent infection of HIV/AIDS among children. UNICEF is also a global leader in vaccine supply, including the hepatitis B vaccine, and reaches 40 percent of the world's children.

### U.S. Centers for Disease Control (CDC)

1600 Clifton Rd.

Atlanta, GA 30333

phone: (404) 639-3311

e-mail: cdcinfo@cdc.gov

Web site: www.cdc.gov

The Centers for Disease Control and Prevention is recognized as the lead federal agency for protecting the health and safety of people at home and abroad, providing credible information to enhance health decisions, and promoting health through strong partnerships. The CDC provides information on the U.S. prevalence rate of STDs, how to prevent getting STDs, what can be done to treat the diseases, and testing and partner notification recommendations.

## U.S. Food and Drug Administration (FDA)

5600 Fishers Ln.

Rockville, MD 20857-0001

phone: (888) 463-6332

Web site: www.fda.gov

The federal agency ensures the public's safety by testing the safety of all drugs, vaccines, medical tests, and medical devices used in the United States. The agency's Web site provides the FDA's assessments of STD treatments and vaccines, including the latest HIV drugs and results of the HPV vaccine trials.

## William J. Clinton Foundation

55 West 125th St.

New York, NY 10027

Web site: www.clintonfoundation.org

Through the William J. Clinton Foundation, former U.S. president Clinton promotes the values of fairness and opportunity for all. The foundation's HIV/AIDS Initiative (CHAI) partners with governments and drug manufacturers to make treatment for HIV/AIDS more affordable and to implement national programs to reach patients in need.

## World Health Organization (WHO)

Ave. Appia 20

CH-1211 Geneva 27, Switzerland

phone: (41) 22 791 2111

fax: (41) 22 791 3111

e-mail: info@who.int

Web site: www.who.int

WHO directs and coordinates all matters related to health within the United Nations. It provides leadership on global health matters, such as STIs and HIV/AIDS. It provides publications, such as *Global Strategy for the Prevention and Control of Sexually Transmitted Infections: 2006–2015*, to help UN member countries plan and lead STI prevention.

# For Further Research

## Books

Jenna Bush and Mia Baxter, *Ana's Story: A Journey of Hope*. New York: Harper-Collins, 2007.

Aine Collier, *The Humble Little Condom: A History*. Amherst, NY: Prometheus, 2007.

Charles Ebel, *Managing Herpes: Living and Loving with HSV*. Research Triangle Park, NC: American Social Health Association, 2007.

Gregory Everson, Hedy Weinberg, and Steve Bingham, *Living with Hepatitis B: A Survivor's Guide*. New York: Hatherleigh, 2001.

Deborah Hayden, *Pox: Genius, Madness, and the Mysteries of Syphilis*. Cambridge, MA: Basic Books, 2003.

Susan Hunter, *Black Death: AIDS in Africa*. New York: Palgrave MacMillan, 2004.

Lisa Marr, *Sexually Transmitted Diseases: A Physician Tells You What You Need to Know*. Baltimore, MD: Johns Hopkins University Press, 2007.

Meg Meeker, *Your Kids at Risk: How Teen Sex Threatens Our Sons and Daughters*. Washington, DC: Regnery, 2007.

Stephanie Nolen, *28 Stories of AIDS in Africa*. New York: Walker, 2007.

Monica Sweeney and Rita Kirwan Grisman, *Condom Sense: A Guide to Sexual Survival in the New Millennium*. New York: Lantern, 2005.

## Periodicals

Lawrence Altman, "Agency Urges a Change in Antibiotics for Gonorrhea," *New York Times*, April 13, 2007.

———, "Sex Diseases Rising: Chlamydia Is Leader," *New York Times*, November 14, 2007.

*American Family Physician*, "Genital Herpes, What You Should Know," October 15, 2005.

———, "Sexually Transmitted Diseases—Prevention and Treatment for You and Your Partner," December 15, 2007.

David Brown, "Pact Would Give Global AIDS Fight Triple the Money," *Washington Post*, February 28, 2008.

Nancy Cibulka, "Mother-to-Child Transmission of HIV in the United States," *American Journal of Nursing*, July 2006.

Staci Dennis, "Worship Service Presented to Increase AIDS Awareness," *Virginian-Pilot*, December 13, 2007.

*Economist*, "And Now Here Is the Virus Forecast," February 21, 2008.

———, "Free to Choose," February 8, 2002.

———, "God, Sex, Drugs, and Politics," February 8, 2007.

David Fine et al., "Increasing Chlamydia Positivity in Women Screened in Family Planning Clinics: Do We Know Why?" *Journal of the American Sexually Transmitted Diseases Association*, January 2008.

Valerie Huber, "Abstinence Works," *USA Today*, July 30, 2007.

*Journal of the American Academy of Physician Assistants*, "The Latest CDC Update to STD Treatment Guidelines," November 2002.

Claudia Kalb and Karen Springen, "The War on HPV," *Newsweek*, May 8, 2006.

Beryl A. Koblin et al., "Hepatitis B Infection and Vaccination Among High-Risk Noninjection Drug-Using Women: Baseline Data from the UNITY Study," *Journal of the Sexually Transmitted Disease Association*, November 2007.

Isadore Rosenfeld, "How to Stay Healthy at College," *Parade*, August 13, 2006.

———, "Let's Help Our Teens Avoid STDs," *Parade*, September 11, 2005.

Lucile Scott, "Native Soul," *POZ*, March 2008.

Steve Sternberg, "Chlamydia Cases Top 1M, While STDs Rise Slightly Overall," *USA Today*, November 14, 2007.

Laura Whitehorn, "What's In, What's Out: A Timeline of HIV Therapy Trends," *POZ*, November 2007.

Lyric Wallwork Winik, "The Test That Could Save Your Life," *Parade*, June 4, 2006.

## Internet Sources

Holly Becker, "Herpes: My Story," Sex, etc., April 18, 2007. www.sexetc.org.

The Body, "Living with HIV/AIDS," June 21, 2007. www.thebody.com.

Andrea Carter, "Condoms Highly Effective Against HPV, Study Shows," ABC News, June 21, 2006. http://abcnews.go.com.

Hepatitis B Foundation, "Hepatitis B Vaccine History." www.hepb.org.

MTV, "It's Your (Sex) Life Guide." www.mtv.com.

Thembi Ngubane, "South African Diary: Living with AIDS," PBS, May 30, 2006. www.pbs.org.

# Source Notes

## Overview

1. Quoted in *Daily Mail*, "The Terrible Price I'm Paying for Teenage Sex," August 31, 2006. www.dailymail.co.uk.
2. Quoted in PBS, "Interview with Raney Aronson: Red Light Reporting?" *Frontline*, June 2004. www.pbs.org.
3. Quoted in *Washingtonian Diplomat*, "New Approaches May Stem Rising Tide of STDs," September 2006. www.washdiplomat.com.
4. Quoted in Avert, "The Impact of HIV & AIDS in Africa," July 31, 2007. www.avert.org.
5. Quoted in Laura Owings, "STDS More Common than Thought," March 1, 2007. http://abcnews.go.com.
6. Quoted in *Economist*, "The Birds, the Bees, and the Taboos," September 13, 2007. www.economist.com.
7. Quoted in Lasker Foundation, "Investment in Research Saves Lives and Money." www.laskerfoundation.org.

## What Are Sexually Transmitted Diseases?

8. Quoted in The Body, "Voices of Hope," July/August 2006. www.thebody.com.
9. Quoted in Sumita Thapar, "When It Comes to HIV, All Women Are at Risk," India Together, December 1, 2003. www.indiatogether.org.
10. Holly Becker, "Herpes: My Story," Sex, etc., April 18, 2007. www.sexetc.org.

## What Are the Dangers of Sexually Transmitted Diseases?

11. Alyson Peel, "Rattling the Gates: A Peace Corps Volunteer's Chronicle of HIV Life and AIDS Death in Swaziland," World Volunteer Web, March 3, 2005. www.worldvolunteerweb.org.
12. Quoted in Mary Robinson, "HIV Positive Women Beaten to Death by Family," International Community of Women Living with HIV/AIDS, February 16, 2005. www.icw.org.
13. Curtis Finney, "Successful Management of Genital Herpes," Herpes.org, February 2002. www.herpes.org.

14. Medscape Today, "Antidepressant Treatment Improves Adherence to Antiretroviral Therapy Among Depressed HIV-Infected Patients," *Journal of Acquired Immune Deficiency Syndromes*, June 1, 2005. www.medscape.com.

## Can Changes in Behavior Prevent Sexually Transmitted Diseases?

15. The United States President's Plan for Emergency AIDS Relief, "Prevention of Sexual Transmission in the General Population," December 2007. www.pepfar.gov.
16. Quoted in Terry Wynn, "Social Issues Linked to Rise in STDs," April 20, 2005. www.msnbc.msn.com.
17. Anne Peterson, "Testimony of Dr. Anne Peterson," USAID, May 19, 2003. www.usaid.gov.
18. Amanda Schaffer, "No More Virginal," *Slate*, April 20, 2007. www.slate.com.
19. Christopher Scipio, "The Ethics of a Lifelong Herpes Infection," Deep Fitness. http://deepfitness.com.
20. Quoted in Michael Shernoff, "Gay Men and Unsafe Safe: Beyond a Knee Jerk Reaction," *Social Work Today*, vol. 3, no. 17, December 2003. www.gaypsychotherapy.com.

## Can Science Eliminate Sexually Transmitted Diseases?

21. Quoted in YOUANDAIDS, "A Life on the Front Line of AIDS Research." www.youandaids.org.
22. Quoted in Edmund Sanders, "New Life for African AIDS Patients," *Los Angeles Times*, February 15, 2008. www.latimes.com.
23. Quoted in PBS, "Interview with Cleve Jones," *Frontline*, May 2006. www.pbs.org.
24. Quoted in Global Campaign for Microbicides, "Quick Quotes." www.global-campaign.org.
25. Quoted in Katha Pollitt, "Virginity or Death," *Nation*, May 30, 2005. www.thenation.com.
26. CDC, "Why Immunize?" July 11, 2003. www.cdc.gov.

# List of Illustrations

Lists of Illustrations

# Index

# About the Author

Leanne Currie-McGhee has written several books for educational publishers. This is her first book for the *Compact Research* series.